The Effortless Power of Kung Fu

Also by Paul Chapman
Stress Proof Your Body
Published by Fairwater Press

Published by
FAIRWATER PRESS

Knowing others is intelligence;
knowing yourself is true wisdom.
Mastering others is strength;
mastering yourself is true power.

Tao Te Ching

Published by Fairwater Press, Reading, England
Email: publisher@fairwaterpress.com
First published by Fairwater Press in 2017
Copyright © Paul Chapman 2017

ISBN: 978-0-9927081-1-5

THE EFFORTLESS POWER OF KUNG FU

A beginner's introduction to the background, training and tactics of Chinese martial arts.

Contents#

Preface   xi

Introduction   1

    A guide to the road ahead   3

    My Background   5

PART ONE – BACKGROUND

Chapter One – What is Kung Fu?   7

    Stop the fight   7

    Four levels   8

    Weapons Training   9

    The yin and yang of kung fu   10

    How kung fu differs from other martial arts   12

    Finding the real knowledge   15

Chapter Two – Functionality in Forms   17

    Stylised forms   17

    Partly functional forms   18

    Fully functional forms   19

    Why adaptability is so important 20

    Forms as a learning aid   20

    Where did the function go?   21

    From forms to formlessness   23

Chapter Three – Sparring and Effectiveness   24

Is sparring proof of effectiveness?   24

Combat variables   25

The four technique variables   27

The YouTube search for proof   28

Technique sparring   29

From forms to sparring   30

Chapter Four – The Rise and Fall of Kung Fu   32

The warrior heritage   33

The Shamanic roots   33

The hundred schools of thought   34

The beginning of Shaolin   34

The vastness of Wudang   35

The end of the Ming   35

Civil war and the Shaolin fire   36

No time to train   37

Standardised kung fu   37

Kung fu's darkest hour   38

The 70s boom   38

The digital age   38

Chapter Five – The Erosion of Kung Fu   40

Learning requires continuity   41

The lack of experimentation   41

The rise of acrobatics   42

Teaching the Confucian way   43

Legends and lineages   44

Chapter Six – Why Learn Kung Fu   47

Balanced training   48

Comprehensive skills   49

Adaptability   51

A strong and healthy structure   52

Chapter Seven – Finding a School   54

Traditional martial arts vs combat sports   55

Belts and gradings   56

What to look for in a teacher   56

The challenges of teaching   58

Kung fu titles   59

The true kung fu Master   60

PART TWO – TRAINING

Chapter Eight – The Basics of Training   63

Generic vs specific training   63

Naming techniques   64

The kung fu body   65

How to train   67

Chapter Nine – Stance Training   70

Horse Stance   73

Dragon Stance   77

Tiger Stance   79

Cat Stance   80

Crane Stance   81

Chapter Ten – Bodyweight Exercises   83

Squats   85

Push Ups   87

Pull Ups   89

Leg Raises   91

The Flying Crane   93

Chapter Eleven – Flexibility and Mobility   96

Why flexibility is king   96

Hard and soft tension   97

Passive and dynamic stretching   98

The Hip and Shoulder Opener   100

The Clock   101

Circular Training   102

Chapter Twelve – Moving with Power   104

A MAP of your training   104

Moving your body   106

Dragon Step   107

Half Dragon Step   107

Half Tiger Step   108

Tiger to Dragon   109

Cat to Dragon   109

Cat Step   109

Chapter Thirteen – Guarding and Blocking   112

    The extended guard.   112

    Yin And Yang Blocks   114

    Yang Circle   116

    Yin Circle   118

Chapter Fourteen – Whole-Body Punching   120

    The mechanics of punching   120

    The dangers of hand conditioning   124

    Iron palm training   125

    Weapons training   126

    Sensitivity training   127

    Dragon Punch   128

    Tiger Punch   130

    Chain Punch   131

    Reverse Chain Punch   133

Chapter Fifteen – Kicking in Real Life   134

    Don't kick high   134

    Front Kick   135

    Back Kick   137

Chapter Sixteen – Effortless Throwing   140

    Taking them down   140

    The groundfighting myth   141

    The three parts to a throw   142

    Dragon Throw   143

    Forward Horse Throw   145

Backward Horse Throw   146

Chapter Seventeen – Connected Power in Kung Fu   149

The two power movements   149

Practice one movement   151

PART THREE – TACTICS

Chapter Eighteen – Gaining Control   153

The rising tide of panic   154

The three types of attacker   155

The three types of martial arts   156

Don't push back   158

Connect and Control   160

Working with a partner   162

The common types of assault   165

Chapter Nineteen – Defences Against Grabs   167

The yin block defence   167

Eagle raises its wings   167

Wrist pull down   168

Defences against grabs from behind   170

Chapter Twenty – Defences Against Strikes   172

Chapter Twenty-One – Defences Against Kicks   175

Chapter Twenty-Two – Defences Against Grapplers   177

Chapter Twenty-Three – Defences Against Multiple Opponents 180

Afterword 182

The 8 animal styles 182

Tiger style 183

Crane style 184

Leopard style 184

Monkey style 185

Eagle style 185

Snake style 186

Mantis style 187

Dragon style 187

Preface

This book is based largely on articles I have written for my online kung fu training website which can be found at www.jadedragonschool.com. Those articles (and accompanying videos) aim to give authentic kung fu training to both the novice and experienced kung fu artist. Kung fu is a vast topic and no matter how long you have studied there is always more to learn. Most, if not all the skills in the book have training videos available on that website and there are more articles and videos being uploaded all the time. Full access to all the material is available for a small monthly fee.

This book is the first book in a series and is based on the Jade Dragon kung fu system. This is the system that I have studied and taught for the last 30 years. It is a little known but comprehensive, traditional kung fu system featuring eight animal styles and a wide range of training practices with both forms and sparring. The eight animal styles are at the heart of the system. There is no space in this book to go into those animal styles in depth, that will be for future books. However, at the end I will give a breakdown of those animal styles and why we study them. The system I know will differ in many ways from other kung fu styles but the basics will be largely the same. The ways of training the body also differ from style to style but what you learn in this book will give you an excellent grounding that you can transfer to other kung fu styles.

I consider myself to be something of a martial scientist. For me, kung fu is about the constant quest to obtain more and more power while using less and less effort. To that end, I am constantly analysing physical structure, tactics, training methods and so on and seeking ways to make them more efficient. As a teacher, I am fortunate to have a wide range of students on whom I can practice and experiment. The Chinese have spent many centuries on this quest and, although some of that knowledge has been lost or destroyed there is no reason why it cannot be brought back through analysis and experimentation. This is largely what this series of books is about. It seems that there are many kung fu schools that understand these principles but don't or can't use them in a martial way and lots of martial arts schools that practice good combat training but are missing many of the principles of efficient body use.

Kung fu is a Chinese art, or family of Chinese arts. To understand kung fu doesn't mean you have to understand or speak Chinese but it is useful to understand a few words as they may have no direct translation into English.

Two methods have been developed to translate Chinese characters into the twenty-six letters of our alphabet. The first system was called Wade-Giles and was used throughout the English-speaking world for much of the twentieth century. The second system is Pinyin. This is the official romanisation system of China and is used by virtually all literate Chinese people. It was developed in the 1950s and is more functional than the Wade-Giles system as it enables any Chinese word to be written in such a way that it can be pronounced by anybody with just a little tuition. However, this book generally uses the older Wade Giles way of romanising Chinese characters rather than the Pinyin system as these words are more familiar to a Western audience. Thus, we have t'ai chi chuan rather than the newer spelling of taijiquan and Taoism rather than Daoism. Occasionally a word is more familiar to a Westerner audience in Pinyin such as qigong (chi-kung in Wade Giles) in which case I have used the more popular spelling. Purists, please don't be offended.

Also in this book, all opponents have been given the male pronoun for ease of use rather than to suggest it is only men who get involved in violent altercations!

One other word on terminology here - the words style and system are often used interchangeably in the martial arts. However, I prefer the word system to denote a collection of styles that share the same principles and practices and are underpinned by a shared philosophy. What I teach is a system of eight styles, each one based on a different animal with differing tactics, movements, and methods of power generation. There is much overlap between them and the principles on which they are based are the same principles you will find in t'ai chi chuan. These are the principles of utmost efficiency of body use. The aim being to use less and less effort to generate more and more power – hence the title of this book. The principles of the Jade Dragon system are largely the same as in t'ai chi chuan but the range of movements and defensive skills we have available is far larger.

A system is a group of styles with the same principles.

For those of you who have studied different kung fu styles you will find much in here you might recognise but you may know it by a different name. Different styles give different names to what are, essentially, the same skills

Apart from being an introduction to kung fu this book aims also to teach you the basics of developing the effortless power that was the hallmark of traditional kung fu. I say was as many of today's kung fu teachings lack this kind of power.

Effortless power means that you have the ability to take on much larger opponents than yourself and manipulate them at will with small and seemingly effortless techniques. I have always been far more impressed by the person who can take a person down and put them in severe pain without hardly moving at all than the one who wastes time and energy with showy, acrobatic skills but achieves little. Modern kung fu is becoming increasingly showy with style being emphasised over content and an emphasis on acrobatics and hyper-flexibility over whole-body power generation and efficiency of movement.

Don't waste your energy on needlessly flamboyant skills.

The emphasis on total efficiency of movement also pays huge dividends to your general health. Learning to stay relaxed under pressure and maintaining good postural and movement habits throughout your life mean that, as you age, your body shouldn't wear out so quickly. Most Westerners are highly stressed and racked with tension and, as a result, they are prone to a wide range of chronic health conditions.

Within this series of books, you will find a range of skills to help you become less tense, calmer and to be able to apply greatly more power and focus to everything you do. This is the real benefit of kung fu training, not the ability to survive a street attack but the ability to survive life with your health and mental faculties intact.

Kung fu is a fighting art but most of the time it is not an external attacker who you are fighting but yourself. You are fighting your old habits, your patterns of tension, your negative thought processes and so on. Kung fu mastery is all about mastery over yourself, not over other people.

Introduction

I believe the ancient and awe-inspiring arts of kung fu had all but completely died out or moved out of China before Bruce Lee was even born. When he wanted to learn kung fu he found many schools practicing what Masters of old called "flowery fists and embroidery kicks". These were movements that looked good but the students didn't have the knowledge or skill of how to use them in combat.

Bruce went on to study wing chun under the legendary Ip Man but when he settled in the US he decided to develop his own style. In the development of his new style Jeet Kune Do he abandoned many of the ways of traditional Chinese martial arts as he found them lacking in realistic combat ability. The two most important elements he rejected were forms and stances.

In this book, we will look at forms and stances, among many other things and see how and why they were so vital to the awesome martial skills of yesterday and why they should still be practiced today. I completely agree with Bruce Lee in that the majority of all forms that are practiced in martial arts schools around the world have very limited combat value. I also agree that almost nobody understands the importance of stance training and its essential role in the development of whole-body power. The fact that Bruce Lee rejected that kind of training means that he didn't fully understand it either.

In this book, you will discover why stances remain the single most important thing for all martial artists to focus on and why forms training, when done properly, is the only real way to teach a martial art.

This book is really an introduction to kung fu - the ancient Chinese system of martial arts that has inspired so many other fighting and self-development arts around the world. Kung fu skills developed and evolved over thousands of years and gradually became highly refined. They were martial in that they were largely used to defend oneself and one's family from attack and art in that they were a way of physically expressing yourself.

At its best kung fu is still the best of the martial arts and not just the martial arts. I believe it offers more in the way of all-round physical, emotional and mental training than any other training or self-development method you could name. Because it offers so much it does take a long time to learn but, to me that is one of its attractions – the fact that it is a path that you can never get tired of. One you can follow for the whole of your life.

Very few people get to see kung fu at its best.

However, I did say 'at its best'. Most people only see the flashy, stylised kung fu that is shown in the movies or in wushu competitions. This is a kung fu that has swapped awesome fighting skill for showy acrobatics. That is a long way indeed from kung fu at its best as I shall explain in due course.

The kung fu of old was more powerful than almost any kung fu today. Good kung fu differs from other martial arts, most noticeably in the way that power is produced. The power that martial Masters of old could produce was awe-inspiring, yet effortless. This power had little to do with the physical size or strength of the practitioner. It has never been about developing specific muscles but about bringing all the muscles to work precisely together. Unfortunately, this essential element of kung fu is often missing in modern kung fu schools. This book, and those that follow, will aim to bring some of that knowledge back into the curriculum of kung fu.

In this book, we will look at what kung fu is and what it isn't. What it used to be and what it has become. We will take a brief but fascinating look at the history of this remarkable art. We will see how it evolved and how it was all but destroyed in the last century. Then we will see why kung fu can be the ultimate art of self-development and self-defence. We'll look at the huge benefits it confers to its practitioners. We'll look at how to find a good school that will help you develop these skills and benefits for yourself. No matter how many books you read they are no substitute for real training with a genuine Master in a good school environment.

Having said that there are some basic skills that can be gained from a book. So, after that we will look at kung fu training and discover a range of exercises to improve not just your physical fitness but your health as well. Finally, we will be looking at some of the uses of kung fu for self-defence and for health purposes. Obviously, it is difficult to learn actual effective techniques from a book as there is no way to adapt the moves or get any feedback as to how well you are learning them. Every part of your body needs to be in the right position for many skills to work at their best and this takes time and good tuition but I'll do my best to give you the basics.

Along the way, you are in for a lot of surprises. I make a lot of assertions in this book, some of them may seem doubtful but all of them have been tested extensively on a wide range of people.

The ancient art of kung fu is dying.

There is little doubt about the slow death of kung fu. There are fewer genuine teachers around every year and fewer students willing to put in the many years of training necessary to scale even the foothills of the art and start climbing towards the peaks. I hope this book inspires a few more people to take the path of kung fu rather than the easier, yet ultimately less rewarding paths of other martial arts.

All around the world kung fu is being side-lined and people are going in droves for other arts such as karate and taekwondo or for MMA type training. Yet these other arts and sports are more limited in their training than good kung fu and the skills they train tend to be more oriented to competitive combat which doesn't necessarily work in the street. They are also very hard to train for those who are in their forties or older. Good kung fu is something you can keep training well into your eighties or beyond.

I do sometimes enjoy watching these combat sports and other martial arts. I always look at them from a tactical point of view. How are they attacking? Are the defences against those attacks effective or is there a better way? You can learn a lot from watching the way other people move and the tactics they use. But remember you can't judge a style by watching a few individuals. The skill levels they are able to show, particularly in sparring are unlikely to represent the highest levels of their art. Also videos, although useful, cannot express what a movement feels like when you are on the wrong end of it. Many movements are far more powerful than they appear in a video and often the people in the videos are accused of 'going with' the movement or faking it when that may not be the case.

Generally, people who want to learn kung fu are looking for quick fighting skills. There are a few of them in this book but kung fu also has thousands more - many more than any other martial art. However, it is the other benefits of kung fu that make people like myself stick with it for decades. Kung fu can be a path without end. A lifetime commitment to the study of endlessly fascinating skills and higher and higher levels of knowledge and self-mastery.

A guide to the road ahead

This book is split into three parts.

Part One covers some background knowledge about kung fu. It covers what kung fu is, what it isn't and how it differs from other martial arts. It discusses the importance of learning forms and also why so few schools teach them well. It talks about the benefits and drawbacks of sparring and how many people believe, sometimes wrongly, that it will give them useful fighting experience. It explores why so few martial artists who learn forms are able to use them successfully in sparring practices.

The book then talks about the rise and fall of kung fu and how it's history ties in with the history of China itself. As dynasties rose and fell so the fortunes of kung fu rose and fell with them. Next, we talk briefly about the reasons why good kung fu is on the decline. These include teachers who are hidebound to their syllabuses and don't experiment, the lack of students who are willing to learn long-term and the reliance of legends and lineages to promote schools. Then we discuss why people still want to study kung fu in the modern world, the myriad benefits of kung fu training - benefits which go above and beyond those of other martial arts. Then we take a look at how to find the right school and teacher for you but be warned this may be the hardest part of all. We'll talk about some Masters I have known who have inspired me to walk this path for so long and the qualities a real kung fu Master possesses.

Let the qualities of true Masters inspire you on your path.

Part Two is the longest section as it covers kung fu training. It covers both generic conditioning for the whole body and specific exercises to train particular skills. There are hundreds possibly even thousands of exercises that have been developed by a multitude of schools in China over the centuries so naturally I can only include a small selection. These are ones that I teach my students and find particularly useful and beneficial.

Much of the training is about developing the 'kung fu body' and we discuss in depth what that is and how to achieve it. Kung fu is a much older martial art and more sophisticated than more modern martial arts in terms of body mechanics and mental focus. In this book, we show some of the real 'secrets' of kung fu training - the real art of generating the truly effortless power that is the hallmark of all good kung fu.

In the third and final part, we discuss the tactics of kung fu. We look at self-defence and the kung fu strategies that should help you survive should you find yourself under threat of attack. Although this section is largely about self-defence it also covers how kung fu is a microcosm of life itself. I am often asked if I've ever used my kung fu skills and the answer is that I use them every day. I use them daily in how I deal with life itself. Decades of training have given me a different perspective on life's large and small traumas. I don't react in the fearful way that others do. I am calmer and more focused. This training makes me more effective and less likely to suffer from the many health issues associated with high stress levels.

Kung fu training brings all the parts of you to work together in a focused way.

Traditionally, kung fu has always had a strong ethical code of behaviour. This is known as wu de. It is a Confucian teaching that exhorts all martial artists to show virtue, honour, trust, respect, courage and justice. Kung fu exists to develop you as a person and not to turn you into a mindless fighter. You learn respect and in learning to respect yourself you also come to truly respect others and the world around you. You discover that, in trusting others you also become more trustworthy and that courage and honour take many forms.

Your martial skill is your sword. It should be taken out frequently and polished (ie practiced) so that it becomes sharp and becomes one with you. When in public it should remain sheathed at all times. Do not feel tempted to show off your skills to others. The blade must not be shown off to anyone unless there is no alternative to actual combat. In which case, it should be used with due respect to yourself, your opponent and to your teachings.

Do not try to practice everything every day. It isn't possible. However, when practicing do so mindfully and not while engaged in other pursuits such as watching the television. Where the mind goes so the intent and energy flows. Also, do not practice while under the influence of drugs or alcohol, while in an angry or otherwise negative mood or when physically or mentally exhausted. All of these things would be detrimental to your health and wellbeing.

My background

I started my journey in kung fu back in the mid-1980s under the little-known Master Irvine in Reading, England. Despite his diminutive size, he is barely over five feet tall, he could throw around guys much larger than me without any apparent effort. Attempting to strike him was also nerve racking as his blocks alone would send pain shooting up your arm. His grabs and locks were excruciatingly painful and I don't even want to think about his strikes. Over the dozen years I studied with him I learned a wide range of animal styles, baguazhang, qigong and meditation. He was not the most approachable of teachers, to put it mildly and like many traditional Masters he spoke little about his personal life or background. However, he could and did perform miracles with casual ease. His fighting skills were extraordinary and on the rare occasions when he would spar with students it was a lesson in sheer terror. Although many students didn't get on with the way he taught none of them had any doubt about his extraordinary commitment and skill level.

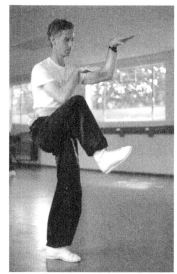

Master Irvine performing snake style

I also studied for a while under Master Zhou in Tunisia (known to his students as Choo Choo). He was another eccentric character but he taught me many valuable lessons including how you could use your mind alone to instantly double the power of your kung fu. This is a skill I will share, in part, later in this book.

For a few years, I became a kung fu wanderer checking out various training halls and Masters and finding a few gems but also a lot of disappointment. I found nobody else who could compare to the Masters who had trained me and realised that such high levels of accomplishment were becoming increasingly rare. I learned that it is far more important to study a single martial art to a high level than to try to learn many different arts with differing practices and principles.

It is better to dig one deep well to find good water than to dig many holes and find only mud.

My original Master gave me permission to teach his knowledge so I set up my own school - the Jade Dragon School in 2003 which I have run ever since. During that time, over 600 students have passed through the doors, some of them briefly but others stayed for many years. In 2013, I wrote my first book 'Stress Proof Your Body' about how to use the principles of kung fu and qigong to reduce tension and so be able to cope better with high levels of stress. This is my second book and I have several more planned.

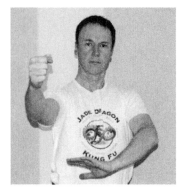

Sifu Paul Chapman

In conclusion, the study of a good martial art is, in my opinion, one of the most rewarding pastimes that one can have. To feel yourself becoming fitter, stronger, faster etc every day is a great boost to one's self-confidence. To know that you have skills that others don't, that you are able to take care of yourself and loved ones should trouble arise, to gradually lose your fears and nervousness of certain situations all of these and many other benefits are yours through gradual, patient and dogged training.

As Lao Tzu so famously said 'A journey of a thousand miles begins with a single step'. If you haven't taken that first step yet then maybe it's time you tried it. If you have then just keep on walking and see just how far you can go.

PART 1 – BACKGROUND

Chapter 1.
What is Kung Fu?

The world of kung fu is vast and mysterious, just like China - the country that created and developed it. Kung fu is known the world over as being a martial art. This is true to a point but it is also so much more than that. Kung fu is not a single martial art as many believe. Instead it has become the generic term for all the many and varied martial arts of China. Kung fu is divided into styles each of which can be very different with different skill sets, methodologies, principles, practices and philosophies. Nobody knows how many kung fu styles are being practiced around the world today but it certainly numbers in the hundreds and is possibly over a thousand. Only a small percentage of these styles have been exported successfully to the West and most Westerners would be hard put to name even a handful of them.

Only a few good kung fu styles are being taught in the West.

Kung fu is a generic term for martial art but it is also a way of life, a pathway to surviving a tempestuous world with your physical and mental health intact. Through your daily kung fu practice you gradually sculpt yourself into a more powerful and less stressed human being.

Within the realms of kung fu lie a vast array of practices to develop the human mind, body and potential to startling degrees. In my, completely unbiased, opinion kung fu is the greatest treasure from the world's oldest civilisation.

Stop the fight

If I had to sum up the purpose of kung fu in just three words those words would be 'stop the fight'. When we think of the word fight in connection with kung fu the natural thought is about physical combat between two or more people. Naturally kung fu gives us skills to bring such a fight to a speedy conclusion. However, we can also use the word fight in a much larger context. The fight is both external towards other people but also internal towards ourselves.

Most people find themselves in internal conflict every single day.

As an example, whenever you tell yourself you cannot do something that you know is expected of you, you are creating conflict inside yourself. This conflict will limit your capabilities and waste your energy while doing so. Kung fu brings about a calmness and purpose of thought that is lacking in most people today. It helps prevent us from getting lost in the endless confusions and indecisions about small things that plagues most people's thought patterns.

Stopping the fight also means preventing your body fighting itself through excess tension that pulls your skeleton in different directions and drains your body of energy. This eventually leads to pain and loss of mobility in later life. The principles of effortless power that you'll find later in this book and in my previous book 'Stress Proof Your Body' help release the tensions that eventually cause so much physical and emotional distress.

Four levels

I was taught from a young age that there are four levels of kung fu but that the vast majority of practitioners never go beyond the first one.

The first level is body: training the body in strength, balance, flexibility, and coordination. Learning to use the entire body together as one unit to generate awesome power with little effort. This book can do no more than introduce you to the basics of the first level.

The second level is breath and energy: learning how to develop a full and balanced breath and then learning how to use that to develop your internal energy, give extra power to your movements, reduce your tension levels and take command of your emotional states. This will be covered in part in future books in this series and is also covered in some detail in my first book 'Stress Proof Your Body'.

The third level is mind: using your mind to create changes in yourself and in your opponent. Again, this will be partially covered later on in this series of books. Only now are we starting to understand the power of the mind to create chemical and genetic changes in our body.

We are, literally, a product of our thoughts.

The final level is universe: becoming completely at one with the circumstances and nature that is flowing around you every second. Acting without the need for thought or resistance or the desire to fulfil other's expectations. Being in the moment and completely at one with yourself and the universe. This goes beyond mindfulness and is the main topic of China's oldest and most fascinating spiritual philosophy - Taoism.

I was fortunate to have two Masters who exemplified and could demonstrate that these aren't airy-fairy fantasies but could genuinely produce awesome, yet effortless power. Not only that but they were no longer tied to forms or set ways of reacting to different threats. This has become the yardstick by which I judge other teachers. They may have fancy looking movements but can they produce awesome power while barely moving and with a calm countenance or a smile on their face? This is real kung fu and it takes a long time to develop.

Kung fu is an endless quest to better yourself.

This is what I love about kung fu. It is a journey without end. Although I now have some of the knowledge of all four levels I know there is still a lot more to learn and discover. In reality, there is no such thing as a kung fu 'Master' as nobody can master all that there is in kung fu. Even in ten lifetimes you couldn't get more than a fraction of it.

Underlying all kung fu training is a set of principles and philosophies. The principles are like rocks on which the training is built. As long as what you are doing follows the principles then it will become effortlessly powerful. The philosophies provide theoretical frameworks which attempt to explain why these kung fu principles work, why we practice them and goes on to examine the human body and mind and its place in the universe.

Weapons training

Weapons training has always been an important part of kung fu. Although the Chinese invented gunpowder they, like the Japanese, shunned the use of firearms in warfare. They believed it dishonourable to use such things and relied on their skills as a fighter to win battles. They developed and used a wide range of bladed and non-bladed weapons and all martial artists would have their own personal weapons that they trained every day and became known for. Hand-to-hand combat was rare in battles, it was only practiced so that you had something to fall back on should you be disarmed. In modern times, this situation has reversed and now firearms and hand-to-hand combat are common whereas the traditional martial arts weapons are no longer used to defend yourself.

The body trains the weapon and the weapon trains the body

The martial artist of old would train his body rigorously to make his weapons use more fluid and powerful. Even the finest sword in the world would be useless in the hands of an untrained person. Equally, the use of the weapon trained the body and the improvement in hand-to-hand skills was a natural extension of the weapons training. Learning to grip and release the weapon improved joint locking skills, focusing your power to the end of the weapon meant you could focus your technique into your opponent's joints to make it more efficient and so on. Although over a hundred different kinds of weapons were developed and used there were four major weapons. Virtually all martial artists were proficient in at least one of these four weapons: the staff, the spear, the broadsword and the double-edged straight sword Often, they would also have their own favourite personal weapon as well which could be anything from a sharpened steel fan to a heavy mace. Each weapon would train the body differently but the goal was always the same – to gain maximum power with minimum effort.

The yin and yang of kung fu

The concept of yin and yang is an important one to understand in kung fu. It is a much misunderstood and underestimated concept. Yet in understanding it you can add great power to your skills.

In China, the symbol we know as the yin yang symbol is called the t'ai chi. The martial and healing art that is based on the t'ai chi is called t'ai chi chuan. The t'ai chi is a symbol that everybody recognises but few people truly understand. When most people talk of t'ai chi they really mean t'ai chi chuan unless they are specifically talking about the yin yang symbol.

The familiar yin-yang symbol, known in China as the t'ai chi

The Chinese of antiquity were very observant. They noticed that everything in nature is changing constantly. They noticed that many of these changes were cyclical. The changing of the seasons, the growth cycles of plants, tidal movements, the cycles of weather and so on. They further noticed that within these changes two specific and complementary forces were at work. They named these forces yin and yang.

In the West, the concepts of yin and yang are sometimes misunderstood which is a shame as an understanding of them explains so much about nature, about movement, about conflict, about the human condition and so much more.

Yin is the force that sinks and contracts. Yang is the force that rises and expands.

The genius of the yin yang (taiji) symbol is that it shows graphically how when one force reaches its zenith then the other force comes into play in a continuous circle. Notice the top of the circle and as the yang (white area) becomes full it starts to become yin (black area). It also shows that nothing in nature is entirely yin or yang, within everything, everybody and every action lies the seed of potential change.

The two forces of yin and yang are at play all around you. Open your eyes and you will see.

- Water evaporates, rises, and expands thus expressing its yang force. Then when it is up in the sky it becomes yin. It contracts and falls downwards as rain. It can then become further yin and harden into ice.

- Spring and summer are yang seasons as life grows and expands then in the autumn and winter (the yin seasons) they contract back into themselves or fall to the earth and die.

- Anger is a yang emotion expanding expressively and forcefully outwards. Sadness, grief, and depression are yin emotions contracting inwards and denying any expression of outward energy.

- Youth is a yang period of life; you grow, express yourself and achieve things. In old age you become yin, you contract into yourself, conserve your energy and meditate.

Yin properties are hard, cold, heavy and tense. Yang properties are the at the other end of the spectrum - soft, warm, light and expressive. This does not mean that yang is, in any way, better than yin. In fact, Taoists tend not to classify anything as good or bad. Within every apparent 'bad' thing lies some 'good' aspect and vice versa.

Anybody who has read more than one book on Taoism, qigong, kung fu or anything of the kind will find that much of the knowledge contained within is apparently contradictory. The concept of yin and yang is seemingly simple, yet it is a concept that seems to be described differently each time depending on who you hear it from or what you read. As an example of this you may often find the quality of hardness described as yang and softness as yin. I have read this in many books yet if you look at yin and yang the way I have described it, which is the way I was taught it, you will find that hardness has to be yin. If coldness is yin then hardness must also be so. Clearly as something gets hotter it also gets softer as the increased heat causes the atoms to vibrate faster. This is the yang force at work creating warmth, expansion, and softness.

Another common misconception, in my view, is the belief that yin and yang are opposites like black and white or male and female. However, this is not really true. They are the two ends of an observable spectrum that is constantly changing from one end to the other. Yin changes to yang and then back to yin in a continuous cycle. Male does not become female and then back to male again. Neither does black gradually change to white in the same way that night (yin) gradually becomes the yang of day and then reverts back to the yin of night-time.

The concepts of yin and yang are extremely important in kung fu as they are in life. Indeed, there is a whole martial art - t'ai chi chuan that is dedicated to an understanding of yin and yang. Generally, in t'ai chi chuan the lower half of the body is yin - sinking down and rooting you firmly to the earth. That is where the real power of the movements lies. The upper body is yang gently rising, expanding and expressing movements. In some movements one side of the body is yin, weighted down and the other is yang, ready to move and express power. Sometimes the whole body may be yin apart from one arm or vice versa. The key to using yin and yang is to recognise which parts of your body in any technique are yin and which are yang and then to exaggerate that element.

Recognise the yins and yangs in your life and work with, not against them

I use the yin yang concept all the time to generate power in my movement skills. To go into the specifics of how that is done is beyond the scope of this book but if you want to learn it properly then I suggest you do what I and countless others have done. Go along to a good, school of t'ai chi chuan. Only there will you come to fully understand how to express yin and yang in your movements and when you have that understanding you can extrapolate that knowledge into your own martial skills. It is definitely worth doing if you wish to fully understand real power.

As you go through this book you will find references to yin and yang. Just remember that yin is sinking and contracting inward and yang is rising and expanding outward.

How kung fu differs from other martial arts

Although there are many different styles of kung fu they tend to have certain similarities. Kung fu has a fluidity that many other martial arts lack. Most of the movements are circular rather than linear which creates a flow from one move to the next. There is no starting and stopping of force but a continuous flow of moves that doesn't cease until the objective has been carried out.

This mirrors the difference between the Chinese and the Japanese cultures. The Japanese mentality tends to be hard and straight as forged steel and they have hundreds of rituals and ceremonies which cover almost every aspect of life. Their martial arts mirror this. They are full of ritual, everything is named and there is a set path from beginner to mastery. Their moves tend to be linear with the philosophy of a straight line being the fastest route from A to B. The Japanese are masters of the straight line where the Chinese are masters of the circle and curve.

In China, nothing is straightforward.

In China, nothing is said bluntly but instead is hinted at in circular ways. Everything is constantly changing so is hard to pin down. In Karate, a Shuto Uke is a knife hand block and couldn't be anything else. In kung fu the same movement could have a dozen or more different uses. Kung fu is more fluid and adaptable to suit changing circumstances than any other martial arts system. I often tell my students that the ability to adapt to change is the most useful thing they learn. This is why kung fu takes longer to learn but the journey is endlessly fascinating.

Kung fu teaches you to remain calm under pressure. Any teacher that promotes an aggressive attitude is not teaching kung fu. The more calm, relaxed and focused you are the more powerfully and effortlessly you can move. It also helps you to deal with high pressure situations such as the threat of attack. You learn not to trigger the 'fight or flight' reflex but to remain calm and keep your mind and body relaxed and ready to respond in the most appropriate way.

Kung fu has a much wider repertoire of techniques than other martial arts.

Judo teaches you to throw but has virtually no strikes or kicks. Conversely karate teaches strikes and kicks but few locks or throws. Within the vast world of kung fu there is every combat skill you can imagine and many more you couldn't. Obviously, none of the many styles of kung fu can teach you all of this - teachers can only pass on skills they know. It is unfortunately true that the skill level and knowledge of the great majority of kung fu teachers is nothing like what it was a century or more ago. Much of the knowledge and skill has been lost and more is being lost all the time. Every time a Master dies without having passed on the full range of his skills some of that knowledge will have died with him. The knowledge should be replaced by existing teachers through experimentation but most of them are so hidebound by tradition that they dare not deviate from their set forms and syllabuses. They don't experiment at all so don't learn anything new. Their knowledge becomes stagnant. It becomes less and less with each generation that passes and eventually dies.

Good kung fu also differs in its tactics from other martial arts. Karate, for example, applies full force in all its techniques where kung fu only uses partial force. A karateka puts his all into each movement - everything is done at full power. A kung fu stylist tends to use only as much force as is necessary to probe his opponent's defences and won't apply anything like full power until he is certain that the technique will succeed. In this way, he conserves his energy and doesn't commit himself and possibly leave himself open until he is sure his opponent cannot counter him effectively. Even when he does attack the way he uses power is more like a dimmer switch than an on switch. At any time, he can change the movement if his opponent doesn't react in the way he expects. This comes only from many years of experience and high levels of skill.

The true essence of kung fu lies in effortless power – the ability to generate great force without straining the body or mind.

It is this effortless power that was experienced first-hand over the centuries by those who attempted to invade the vast land of China. The Mongols, Manchus and Japanese, among others, all faced skilled kung fu fighters in combat and were amazed at the effortless power that they could command. But without knowledge of the training practices they used to develop this power the invaders sought to emulate and develop it using physical strength instead.

The real effortless power of ancient kung fu isn't achieved through weight training or calisthenics although these can be useful, but through an understanding of a connected physical structure. With this structure comes physical power and skill that is out of proportion to the practitioner's size. This type of power is rarely apparent in other martial arts. Some, like aikido and judo have a taste of it but the way they develop the structure differs from good kung fu. In kung fu every part of you comes together in a focused way to create the power. The skeleton is precisely aligned with the forces acting on it, only the muscles needed are engaged in the movement and all other muscles are relaxed, the breath powers the body from the inside and the mind is totally focused on the skill in hand. I will teach the basics of the practice later on in this book.

I should point out that there are two main types of kung fu training. I call these yin and yang. Yang kung fu is the showy, acrobatic kung fu that focuses on mobility and flexibility and is the kind you will be most familiar with. The other way is yin kung fu. This focuses on connected, whole-body power and efficiency of movement. These are sometimes referred to as internal (yin) kung fu and external (yang) kung fu. This book is mostly based on yin kung fu training which, in my opinion, is the better kind. This is the healthiest type of training and will keep you strong and mobile well into your old age.

Finding the real knowledge

We live in a marvellous age. A world's worth of information is available with a few clicks of a mouse. We are now able to gain knowledge and insights in a few moments that would previously have taken years to achieve or may never have been possible. In other words, information is now cheap.

Anybody who studies the martial arts, particularly the Chinese martial arts will find a huge wealth of information to help them further their understanding of their art. There are thousands of books, YouTube videos, blogs and so on to help them understand areas that may not be fully covered in the classes they go to. Unfortunately, much of the information is conflicting. If for example you wanted more information about fajin or iron shirt or breathing exercises or specific striking methods etc. you would find many different methodologies, principles, and exercises from a variety of sources, all of them claiming to be genuine and effective. How do you know what is the right and most effective way to do things?

The short answer, unfortunately, is that you can't. These skills were developed in times of necessity when your fighting skill kept you and your clan alive. A huge number of ways of turning a human being into an efficient fighter have been developed throughout history all around the world though it's generally accepted that the most sophisticated of these skills were developed in the Far East, particularly in China.

The Chinese people have a long history of combat, whether against rampaging warlords, invaders from outside or the armies of the emperor. The need for martial skills has been necessary for at least 3000 years. China is both a vast country and also very insular. Most Chinese people never travelled far, extensive travel within China was rare apart from for traders. China is a country so insular that people from neighbouring villages can talk completely different languages. Unlike today there was little real communication between the various parts of the Chinese empire so different martial arts grew up independently with differing skills sets, training methods and philosophies.

Imagine if you suddenly found your home being raided by fighters from another village. You fought well using the skills your family had developed but you found that the strikes you had worked so hard to develop were just bouncing off them and weren't injuring or killing them as you'd imagine. Clearly, they had developed a method to withstand your strikes. How did they do that? They will be paranoically possessive of such skills and are certainly not going to teach it to you so you need to work out your own methods for achieving the same effect.

In this way, the same skill gets developed at different times and places with the same, or similar effect being achieved through different methods. Which is the best method? Nobody knows or can know until such things can be scientifically tested. Many schools claim that they developed their skills themselves and that their way is the best.

This is why we have so many different methods for so many different skills that achieve the same or similar result. This is why we have such a plethora of books and videos and nobody can say for sure which is the best way to do anything. This is both good news and bad for the serious student of these arts. You can never know that the methodology you're practising is the best one for you. It may have been the best way for the person who developed it but they aren't you. The good news is that even if, despite your best efforts, you aren't making progress after a reasonable length of time there will always be another methodology out there.

This is also the reason why we have arguments about who founded this art or developed that skill. A good example is the ongoing debate about who founded t'ai chi chuan. Some believe that the art was founded by a Taoist monk called Zhang Sanfeng in the twelfth century. Others say that it was started by the Chen family who claim that they developed the art in the seventeenth century.

The idea of using relaxed power and efficient body use to develop the internal energy for fighting would have been one that almost certainly occurred to more than one person. Arts and skills based on these principles were given a variety of names until the name t'ai chi chuan was arrived at in the mid nineteenth century.

I find it entirely possible that the principles that t'ai chi chuan is based on were developed independently with differing movements and methods. After all, t'ai chi chuan is based on well-known Taoist principles and employs utmost efficiency of body use as an overriding goal. These are principles that most martial artists would aspire to. It only required some training in Taoist philosophies and meditation practices to discover these principles independently. After that, of course, would come years of experimentation to nail down the most effective methods.

Many discoveries, inventions and principles are discovered or invented by several people independently and separately.

This is known as multiple discovery. The list of multiple discoveries is long and includes the invention of the telephone, calculus, the discovery of oxygen, the theory of evolution of the species and so on. Each of these was discovered or invented independently by more than one person often within a short time of each other. To me what matters is not so much the background of what you are studying or who invented it, which you can never know for certain but the principles and practices that it entails. These are what will provide the results you seek not the often-mangled history behind it. Anyway, it is not beyond the realms of possibility that t'ai chi chuan developed independently in more than one place. Of course, we can never know for sure but it's a theory and may help these battling t'ai chi families find harmony with one another.

Chapter 2.
Functionality in Forms

Martial arts schools can be classified in many ways. One way is whether the school is focused more on learning forms or on sparring. Both methods of training have their advantages and their place but there are few schools that do both successfully. Most schools that teach forms aren't able to use the movements from their forms (known as katas in Japanese styles) in their sparring. So, what are forms and why do they seem to be increasingly useless in combat?

In this chapter, we will look at the three main types of forms training and how forms training is gradually degenerating from being the most efficient way to learn and develop real, adaptable fighting skills into competitive, stylised dance movements with little or no combat capabilities. The article focuses strongly on Chinese martial arts which is the focus of this book but the concepts are the same no matter which martial art you study.

A form in Chinese martial arts is a series of movements that is designed to teach a set of martial skills and exercise the body in a wide variety of ways.

Learning forms has been the most effective way of passing on martial arts knowledge for many centuries. A form may be focused on learning a particular type of movement such as kicking forms, or on a weapon such as staff forms or just on more general skills. Usually the more advanced the form is, the more specialised the movements are. Basic forms may teach a variety of fundamental skills where advanced forms focus on a specific type of skill such as attacking nerve endings with fingertip precision. Most modern forms taught in kung fu schools now range from stylised forms through partly functional to the much rarer fully functional forms. This article examines the differences.

Stylised forms

A stylised form is a series of movements of stylised fighting skills. These forms are characterised by beautiful, acrobatic movements. The form is judged on how it looks and how precisely it is performed. The form is taught exactly the same way every time and gradually the practitioner is able to perform the movements with more grace and skill, going lower in the stances, becoming more flexible in the kicks and so on. However, despite the beauty of the form the applications are missing. Students aren't taught how to use these forms for fighting. It is 'art' but it has lost the 'martial' quality.

These forms are common in wushu and many t'ai chi schools and, indeed many kung fu forms are of this type. If the form you are learning is being done the same way every time, if you are being judged on the way it looks rather than on how it can be applied, if you are not being shown any fighting applications or being given any chance at partner practice to see how it works then it is a stylised form. These forms are common simply because they are easy to teach and to learn. No instruction on how to adapt the movements or how to use the skills under real life situations are needed.

In China, stylised forms were often taught to children to develop strong stances, joint flexibility, fluidity of movement and so on. Acrobatic movements were often introduced to keep children interested and develop their muscles in explosive movements. Then as they became older the forms would change to become more focused on developing whole-body power. These children's forms are now being taught to adults and being promoted as being good, traditional kung fu. They are nothing of the kind. They are a modern dance that resembles the skills of ancient China, but are little more than a beautiful snake that's had its venom drawn.

Partly functional forms

With partly functional forms the teacher will know some applications for the form but not the full knowledge of how each movement works and how to adapt it to suit changing circumstances. I often see students who have learned forms elsewhere but have little or no idea how to use them. A partly functional form could be anything from knowing just one or two applications to knowing the main applications for each movement. However, partly functional forms are missing the inner moves and how to adapt them. If your teacher only knows one application per movement then it's a partly functional form. Each movement of a fully functional form would have many ways in which it could be applied, not just one.

Learning partly functional forms can be dangerous. You are taught that these are combat skills but if you try to use them in the street and your attacker doesn't react in the way you expect, which is likely, you will be in big trouble. If you aren't instantly able to adapt those movements to the way your attacker has reacted you could be in for something of a rude awakening.

Partly functional forms, like stylised forms, tend to be done much the same way every time. They lack the complete adaptability of fully functional forms. This makes them only partially useful at best. They could be said to be 'martial' but lacking the 'art' element which makes them changeable and expressive.

Fully functional forms

Functional forms don't look anywhere near as beautiful as stylised forms. Good kung fu wasn't developed to look pretty. Truly functional forms may not be good to look at but they do still contain obvious grace, balance, and power. The difference is that every single movement, indeed the smallest part of each movement is functional. The teacher knows all his movements inside out and can adapt and apply every single movement to a range of real fighting applications. He knows where each part of the body should be for every movement and why it needs to be there. He also knows, and is able to teach the students how to make each movement as powerful and efficient as it can be under pressurised circumstances.

The other main difference is that the functional form is completely changeable and adaptable. Every aspect of it: the depth of the stances, the position of the hands, the size and direction of the circular arm movements, the direction of the stepping movements, which stances are being used and when etc are all fluid and changeable.

Only by being completely adaptable to the constant changes that take place in combat can any form be of use in real combat.

A functional form that is truly 'alive' will almost never be performed in exactly the same way twice. It becomes a way of expressing yourself through your body, your movements and your art – indeed it is what puts the word art into martial arts. There is no more 'right way' to do a functional form as there is a 'right way' to paint a tree. It depends on the circumstances. There are, however, many wrong ways. These will be the ways where the body is being used ineffectively or the technique being applied doesn't fit with what the opponent is doing. This ability to be able to read your opponent and adapt your techniques accordingly – to be able to express yourself through your movements, prevents your martial arts from becoming too rigid which would mean you've lost the art in your art form. By constantly changing the way that you perform your movements during solo practice you remain constantly open to change and the possibility of adaptability.

In order to be sure that your functional form is truly functional it must be tested against resisting opponents against a wide range of attacks. This is something that is built up gradually. You start with slow, predictable attacks then slowly make them harder to defend against. You must use your form movements, keeping to all the principles of whole-body power and adapting them as you go to the attacks that come your way. This has been likened to playing chess at high speed and is where forms training meets sparring practice. Nowhere near enough kung fu schools pressure test their forms properly which is why they can't use them in sparring. A newcomer to kung fu would have thought it obvious and logical that this should be done but it rarely is.

Why adaptability is so important

When you perform any movement on any resisting opponent you have no idea how that opponent is going to react. They may fall to the floor, they may stand up and resist fiercely, they may step forward on a different leg than you were expecting, they may attack with a different arm etc. If you can't instantly adapt your movement skills to the change then you will probably lose. All the movements of a good, functional form should be doing the following:

1. Protecting your body from attack not just from your opponent but as far as possible from other directions as well through continuous twisting movements that keep you aware of movement from any direction.

2. Doing movements that limit what your opponent is able to do next so that you can predict their likely next moves and already be in a position to take advantage of them. For example, by blocking an attacking arm and leading it down low you know the other arm will have to come over the top so it becomes a predictable response.

3. Keeping you constantly alert and adaptable to how your opponent is reacting to your technique so that, no matter what the opponent does, you can follow them, see and feel the weaknesses in their movements and exploit them ruthlessly.

4. Training your body to move as one unit in the most efficient and powerful ways possible.

5. Teaching you an encyclopaedic knowledge of techniques that can be applied through the movements of the forms. Any movement of the form could easily have ten or more different ways of applying it. Through learning this knowledge, you learn which technique to attempt at any moment depending on your position relative to that of your opponent.

Forms as a learning aid

Forms are the main way of enabling students to memorise a wide variety of techniques.

Learning a martial art is like learning a new language. You don't start at the letter A and work through the alphabet. You start by talking in simple sentences and build them up to tell stories. Good forms have been used for centuries to teach a wide variety of martial skills. It's just like learning to converse in a new language – your opponent makes a movement, you see it, interpret it and come back with an appropriate reply. Your reply is one that allows only a limited set of responses from your opponent and you learn how to reply to each of those responses. If they respond in an unexpected way your form should be adaptable enough to cope without leaving you hesitating and getting hit while you think of an appropriate response.

Your techniques are the words of the sentence. The principles of effective movement are the letters that make up the words. There are only so many principles but on those few principles stands thousands of techniques. Without the principles, your words will have no impact. The forms are the stories you learn that express the art of your style. The art lies in choosing the right words for the occasion while under extreme pressure. Basically, learning forms by repeating them exactly the same way every time is like painting by numbers. Eventually you have to move past and adapt your skills to express your art more fluidly.

Where did the function go?

It is worth saying that most stylised forms used to be fully functional. Unfortunately, due to various reasons including political interference, wars, not allowing outsiders access to the secrets that keeps their clan alive etc the Masters of old decided to hide the secrets of how to use their form movements for fighting.

Instead they developed their forms into ones that were good exercise for the body but had little, if any, practical applications or if they did have practical applications they were hidden within the movements. The form movements became a way of training the body correctly and if you understood the system you would know how to use these skills for real. However, if you just copied the movements without being trained how to use them it would be very difficult indeed to extract the real combat skills from them. These new stylised forms enabled the Masters of old to maintain their movement skills but without overtly displaying the functional combat skills hidden within them. Hence only the Master and his most senior students would be able to interpret the form and be able to fully use all its applications.

It takes a lot longer to learn and master forms that are adaptable. You learn the basic movements which are like a skeleton and then you learn to adapt it endlessly depending on how your opponent reacts to it. This ability to be sensitive to your opponent's actions and constantly be adapting your form movements to it takes time and experience. It is much easier to teach somebody a set series of movements that doesn't change.

This is the main reason why set forms (stylised or only partly functional) are often taught in large schools. It is much easier for a small school with a small number of students to teach a fluid, adaptable form than for a large school which probably has a more rigid syllabus and would find it far more difficult to teach and grade such adaptable forms.

Many modern martial artists denigrate the teaching of forms (the most famous critic being Bruce Lee). They have no place in the real world they say. They lack realism, they aren't tested against a resisting partner, they are too fancy, during sparring practice everyone abandons the forms and just kicks and punches – they just don't work in the ring or on the street. These detractors are absolutely right if they're talking about stylised forms. It may well be only stylised forms that these detractors will have seen because they are far more common than fully functional ones. Also, it is difficult to show fully functional forms as they don't look too good when done on their own and even experienced martial artists wouldn't see most of the applications within them. You really need to experience them first hand. Yet those forms have one main aim in mind and that is to put the opponent at a major disadvantage right from the start and deny them the ability to counter successfully while attacking from a bewildering range of directions with differing types of attack.

The number of teachers who are currently able to teach good fully functional forms is decreasing rapidly.

Forms teaching is becoming increasingly stylised and that is the reason why, I believe good kung fu is dying out. When the teachers have lost the inner meanings and applications of their forms it is incredibly difficult for them to be found again. Without the knowledge of how to use the movements properly, the way the movements will be performed will drift further and further away from being functional and will be focused instead on looking aesthetically pleasing.

It is inevitable that if something has no function that it be made to look beautiful instead.

In the Jade Dragon school, which is a small school, all our forms are fully functional and will always remain that way, indeed I often look at form movements that students have learned in other schools and show them how to make those movements work for real. The most common phrase I hear is "why did nobody teach me this before?" Why indeed.

Forms are a necessary stepping stone in the learning process. You learn the form, you extract from it all that it can offer. All the exercise potential, all the applications and the many ways they can be adapted, all the ways in which it can teach you to move and generate power should be taken from the form. When you have this knowledge, you can keep practicing the form and try to develop and evolve the form further or move onto learning a new and higher-level form. Some forms are fairly basic and teach low level skills. These were often taught to children in China yet many of these forms are now being taught to adults in the West who believe they are learning something special. They never learn to evolve these forms so their own development is limited to the potential of the form.

In my school, I know many different versions of the forms. I take my students through different stages of development. When they absorb one movement and technique then I refine it and make it more sophisticated so they don't lose interest.

From forms to formlessness

At the end of the day, once you have learned what you need from the forms you don't need to practice them anymore. After all, when you were learning to read as a child, you did so by learning stories. That doesn't mean you have to keep reading the same stories every day otherwise you'll forget how to read! It is the same with kung fu. You go beyond forms to formlessness. Your aim is to be completely malleable with each movement perfectly matched to the circumstances of combat. If you are tied to any form it will limit what you can do. This is also where your kung fu movements become a perfect physical expression of yourself. The ability to be able to physically express yourself in any way you choose is so powerful. This is what puts the art into martial arts. This is the Taoist way. In my humble opinion, it is the most fulfilling and enriching experience you can have.

Chapter 3.
Sparring and Effectiveness

When people think about kung fu they think about fighting. When people think about fight training they think about sparring. Many people believe that sparring is good training should you find yourself in a fight. To a certain extent I agree but it partially depends on how you spar and this chapter will explain what I mean.

There are hundreds of styles of martial arts being practised in the world today and thousands of martial techniques. Which of these are the most effective and how can we prove that? The internet forums and social networking sites are alive with arguments and counter arguments claiming all kinds of things while others just as passionately refute them. Many claim for evidence of some kind to 'prove' that such a technique would work for real against a resisting opponent, but what evidence is there?

We live in an age where videos can be quickly and widely disseminated. There are thousands of YouTube videos showing martial arts training and applications which are hotly disputed as to their efficiency and veracity. It is true that only a few of these show techniques being used against a moving or resisting attacker. Most videos show a martial artist performing a technique against a compliant arm being waved in their direction and naturally these are seen as 'not proof' that such a technique would work against someone who really fought back. However, the only thing that can be logically taken from that is the statement below.

If a technique cannot be made to work against a non-resisting attacker then it won't work against a resisting one.

Is sparring proof of effectiveness?

Many martial artists are saying online that the only proof that a move would work for real in a real-life setting is if it worked in sparring. This is a fallacy. Always remember the following.

If a technique doesn't work in sparring all it means is that you couldn't get it to work against that particular person at that particular time under those particular circumstances. Somebody else may be able to get it to work. It may work under different circumstances (see the list of variables below). It may work against a different opponent but not this one. We are all built differently and each person will react differently to everything you do. Some of these will be trained reactions and some will be natural to that person's body type.

Combat variables

The point about sparring is that the variables involved in two people in any combat situation are huge. These variables mean that some techniques may work and others you may struggle to get to work effectively. That doesn't mean that the technique should be abandoned but that it may well work under different circumstances.

Here are just a few of those variables:

1. The fighting skill set you possess

2. Your reaction speed

3. Your attitude, fitness and health level

4. The fighting skill set of your opponent

5. The reaction speed of your opponent

6. The health and fitness level of your opponent

7. The rules of engagement

8. The environment of engagement - including any safety gear you may be using or wearing

9. The four technique variables of distance, angle, timing and contact.

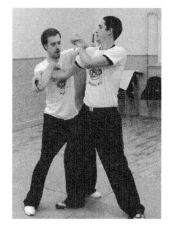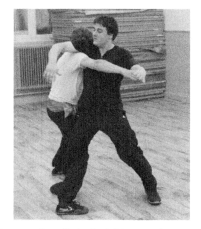

Students vying for an advantage in sparring. Note that this sparring
doesn't involve protective equipment.

Each of these variables limits your number of usable techniques.

- If you possessed every fighting skill on earth you'd have a vast range of skills to call on but you don't. You only have those you've learned and trained well enough to do under pressure. When you're under attack often the mind goes blank and you forget the majority of the skills you've learned. Often you can only remember barely a handful and so you struggle to apply them successfully. There will be other skills you know but not well enough to do them in a sparring situation with success. This could be increased through good, functional forms training but it rarely is.

- Reaction speed is clearly critical. Things happen in milliseconds in combat. Opportunities appear then disappear again and you need to stay in the moment to take advantage of any small gaps in your opponent's defence before they're gone.

- Your attitude, fitness and health level can severely limit how much speed and power you can use at that moment and how quickly you can react to changing circumstances. Attitude is particularly important. Often the one who most believes they will win do so.

- Your opponent's fighting skill set may be larger or less than yours. Only prolonged sparring will really show the limits of each other's knowledge and where you may be at an advantage or disadvantage.

- In sparring you will almost certainly be up against your classmates. People you know and who have trained to fight the same way that you have. This means that you can, to a large degree, predict what they're going to do and how they're going to react. Clearly this isn't the case out there in the real world.

- Your opponent's reaction speed may be faster than yours. He can then manipulate you by being more in control of himself and the situation.

- Your opponent's level of health and fitness may limit his abilities and give you an edge. Or vice versa.

- The rules of engagement will limit the number of techniques available as some may be deemed illegal. Clearly there are no rules on the street. This is where many sport martial arts fail as they aren't trained to defend against certain 'illegal' techniques. It is worth learning the illegal moves of different combat sports as people who participate in those sports won't be trained to defend against them.

- The environment will play a major part in what is possible. Is it a crowded bar or are you in a controlled ring environment? What are you wearing? Tight jeans limit leg use, certain types of gloves limit grabbing movements and so on. Again, this is a potential weakness of combat sports as you are fighting in a controlled environment one man against one man. This is very rare in real life where many attacks involve more than one attacker and the environment can change quickly.

The four technique variables

Distance

Virtually all martial techniques work best at a specific distance from the opponent. Grapplers can't really work at kicking distance and vice versa. Good use of footwork should bring you and keep you at a good distance for the style of combat you prefer. Good martial arts schools will teach a range of skills that can be applied from all distances as well as foot and arm work that will help you get the distance and angle you need.

Angle

Similarly, certain skills only work well at a particular angle to an attack. Throws are a good example of this. These can be hard to get on a moving target and are usually preceded by other moves that limit the opponent's next moves and allow you to predict their response. Then you may find the angle you need to get a particular technique to work. Usually though it just happens by being alive to what's going on and if you see the angle you need you take advantage of the opportunity to try that technique.

Timing

Timing and speed go hand in hand but it's not about how quickly you can move. It's about how well you can match the speed of your technique to your opponent's speed. If you're too quick or too slow you've lost that opportunity. Sometimes, for example, you need to wait for them to change direction then follow them and add power of your own. Also, and perhaps more importantly is moving at a speed that enables your whole body to move as one integrated whole. Commonly when under pressure the upper body moves faster than the lower body and this severely limits how much power can be applied in a movement skill.

Contact

A lot of training in certain martial arts such as t'ai chi chuan and wing chun revolves around maintaining physical contact with your opponent. Sticking hands, push hands, chi sau, rou shou and so on all train you to follow your opponent's moves to maintain contact. With physical contact, you can feel what they are doing and redirect their force. You can react to touch much faster than you can react to what your eyes can see. However, as soon as you lose that contact you lose that control over the situation and again have to rely on your eyes and hope that your reactions will be fast enough. Of course, it goes both ways as you can both feel and redirect attacks equally so then it comes down to who is the most sensitive, has the fastest reactions and most skill in other words the other variables then come into play.

Don't misunderstand me, I like sparring. It has a valid role to play in any martial arts training. It helps to develop confidence, timing, positioning and aggressiveness. Over the last thirty plus years I have sparred with dozens, perhaps a hundred or more people with a wide range of martial backgrounds and skill levels. One of the main things I have learned is that you cannot focus on getting any particular technique to work in sparring. You can only stay in the moment, keep your defences up and take whatever opportunities present themselves. Some techniques will work with some types of attacker (dare I say who have learned certain styles and ways of moving) and some won't. Never forget, you cannot force a technique into a situation but should just allow the situation to dictate the skill or technique. Having said that it is good to practice a few techniques and know them inside out. You should be able to apply them to a wide range of resisting partners under many different circumstances. You may have many skills but these are the ones that will stand you in good stead in a real fight.

In conflict, you must perform your skills under great duress and their effectiveness depends on the reactions of an unpredictable opponent.

I suspect that a lot of traditional schools don't spar very much, or indeed at all. I hear this a lot from students who have come from other schools. If it is true then it's a shame as you can learn so much from sparring. Maybe it's the teachers who are scared of losing to their students with the loss of reputation that would imply. Maybe it's the thought that the techniques they teach are hard to apply in a moving combat situation. But that can be said of any technique. A hint to those who do spar and are struggling to get specific techniques to work is to look at the four technique variables of timing, angle, distance, and contact. Often, it's not the technique itself that doesn't work but it's getting into the place where you can make it work. It's the movement or two before the technique that dictates whether a technique is possible or not. Functional forms training teaches you not to rely on specific techniques but still to follow the skeleton of the form's movements and adapt them to the changing winds of combat.

The YouTube search for proof

Those who are looking for 'proof' of whether certain skills work or not often look to YouTube videos to find examples of techniques working on resisting opponents. As I've mentioned there are so many variables in sparring and things happen so quickly that any technique that works well is as much down to luck as anything else. Nobody could get a technique, any technique to work consistently on a wide range of people in sparring. Once you've got it to work once your opponent knows about it and knows to look out for it and counter it or adapt to it.

There are nowhere near as many sparring videos on YouTube as there are demonstrations of techniques done against a non-resisting attacker. It's not easy to look good when sparring. It's much easier to look impressive when you can control every part of your movement and can show off your amazing skills at being able to defend yourself against a fist that's being waved vaguely in your general direction. And as there are so few good sparring videos it is indeed hard to find 'evidence' that a particular technique could work.

The fact that there are so many negative comments attached to every martial arts video on YouTube has put a lot of people off from posting anything at all on there. It's hardly surprising. Videos can show a certain amount but they are only taken from one angle and are very bad at showing the amount of real power that some moves have. Often people are accused of going with a move or overreacting when that may not be the case. It's often impossible to tell. As an example, often my students will, to a certain extent, go with a technique I'm doing to them simply because it's too painful not to.

YouTube videos are nothing more than a moment frozen in time that gets endlessly debated over.

So much of real martial arts training isn't about what you can see but what you can feel and no video can get anywhere near replicating that hence the endless debates and comments about whether this or that really works.

Technique sparring

As a final convincer to show you that it is extremely difficult to get any particular technique to work in sparring you could try what we do in our school. We call it technique sparring. The idea is simple. You think of a technique you know well and try to apply it to your partner (without telling them what it is). In the meantime, of course, they are trying to apply their own favourite technique on you. We have tried this many times and not once has anyone actually managed to get any technique to work properly under those circumstances. The only conclusions you can draw from this are either: no techniques work in sparring or more likely it's not worth focusing on any specific techniques in sparring but just go with the flow.

From forms to sparring

It is certainly true that many kung fu practitioners cannot use their form movements in sparring. They end up using basic kicks and punches like anybody else. This isn't necessarily a fault of their forms but the fact that they don't have a way to progress their forms into genuine sparring practices.

To turn form movements from solo practice into ones that can be performed in sparring requires several steps. You must train with non-resisting partners first then gradually make the partner's attacks less consistent and with more resistance. You must learn to change your form movements to suit the attacker and the way he is attacking. All the time while doing this you must keep to the principles of whole-body power which are critical in getting your form movements to work.

With consistent practice, you should be able to get your form movements to work most of the time against a range of attackers. Over time you will gain the experience to know that if a movement cannot be made to work then it can instantly be changed to one that will. Never try to force a movement to work if it doesn't work straightaway. Adapt it to suit the attack or abandon it completely and try a different move or tactic.

In combat, it often isn't survival of the fittest but survival of the most adaptable and the one with the most will to win.

One final word on sparring – leave your egos at the door. As I mentioned earlier I have sparred with a great many people and, indeed am happy to cross hands with anyone. But when I do so it is always in the spirit of enquiry, in the spirit of 'what can this person and I learn from each other and this particular sparring session'. At no point is either party trying to 'win' the sparring session or to make the other person feel stupid. Instead of focusing on winning you should be thinking 'This is a new person in front of me. He may move in ways I'm not used to. He may have different tactics and techniques than I've dealt with before. How well can I adapt my defences and attacks to fit in with his.' By thinking along these lines, you aren't investing your ego in the outcome and are truly learning from the experience.

The way forward

To summarise the last two chapters, if you wish to learn a genuine martial art then you need to make your forms functional. The first stage is perhaps the most difficult. You need to learn the combat applications of your forms, but this may not be easy to do. The applications may be hidden or, over time the movements have moved away from the original combat applications. It may require a lot of experimentation to understand their meaning and get them to work consistently. This is a job for the teacher but he can and really should do so through experimentation with his more senior students.

The second step is adaptation. When the applications are workable in how many different ways can you adapt them? Can a punch become a throw or a joint lock? Can a block and lock of the right arm be applied to the left arm without changing it? You may well find that the moves work equally well no matter what kind of attack you face. You will just find that the result differs. Your opponent may go down on his front instead of his back or will drop to his knees instead of turning away from you or something like that. You cannot accurately predict how anyone will react but the next move of your form should be ready to meet the most likely counters or reactions to your previous move.

Once you have identified the applications and can adapt them to the changing winds of combat your next step is pressure testing. As mentioned earlier, this is done initially with predictable attacks and then against increasingly unpredictable ones.

Never forget, you can't ever rely on getting any technique or form movement to work consistently in sparring or real-life conflict for a variety of reasons. But, the more form movements you know that you can get to work under pressure the more chance you have of being able to deal successfully with whatever an opponent may throw your way.

Chapter 4.
The Rise and Fall of Kung Fu

To really understand kung fu it helps to understand the history behind it. Kung fu developed over a vast area over a very long period of time. This is why the styles and practices of kung fu are so varied today. Although China has had written records for longer than any other civilisation there is much dispute about many aspects of kung fu history. There are hundreds of legends and stories which may be pure myth or only partially true. This is particularly true when it comes to the more famous Chinese arts and none more so than the legends surrounding the kung fu of Shaolin and the origins of t'ai chi chuan. No history can claim to be definitive. Bear that in mind as you read on.

Like China, the country that spawned it, kung fu has a long history and is replete with legends about heroic Masters who were humble in life and invincible in combat. To be honest these legends have never held much interest for me. Each culture has its legends of historical heroes. I am far more interested in what skills a person can show me today rather than what some legend who supposedly trained in their school could do some five to ten generations ago. However, many schools base their reputation on these legendary folk heroes. To me this is a mistake and one I shall go into later.

The history of the martial arts of China is interwoven with the history of the country itself. China has a turbulent past and no period was more turbulent than the twentieth century. Throughout Chinese history as emperors and regimes rose and fell the traditional martial schools were either encouraged or under attack.

The kung fu schools have always been a threat to the Government of the day.

It is completely understandable that the ruling classes viewed the traditional schools with suspicion. If you were a Chinese emperor you would have an imperial guard of fiercely loyal and highly trained warriors. Yet you would be ever aware that, in the vast country you ruled, there would be schools and individuals with skills that may well be superior to those of your own army. If enough of these schools banded together they could prove a real threat to your own safety as emperor and to the stability of the realm at large.

It is for that reason that, for many periods of history, the martial arts were forbidden to be trained and the schools were forced to train in secret. But let's go back to the beginning to see how the arts grew and developed.

The Warrior Heritage

Martial arts have been developed and refined in China for many thousands of years. China has over 4000 years of written history and is perhaps the world's oldest surviving civilisation.

For much of its history, China has been filled with internal strife. There have been many warlords trying to gain control of certain areas, invasions by foreign hordes and fragmentation of political control. All of these along with the constant threat of bandits has meant that, for the Chinese, their safety, even their very survival could well depend on their skills as a warrior.

The Shamanic Roots

The story of martial training in China almost certainly began long before any forms of writing were developed. We can never know what were the first types of combat to be trained and used. However, the skills that were learned and refined were enormously valuable and would have been passed on orally and through specific training within a family or clan. The oldest Chinese writings that have been discovered show many martial arts concepts and skills. These were carved into bone and tortoiseshell. There have

also been found many axes, spears and swords of surprisingly high quality which are as much as 7000 years old.

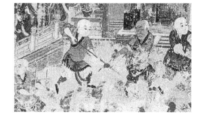

Any implements, rocks, clubs, tools and so on that could be used as a weapon would most likely have been experimented with and then trained as part of the warrior's skill set. Many of these young schools took their combat inspiration from the natural world around them. Movements and tactics would have been developed from strong weather patterns such as storms and tornadoes, from the power of moving bodies of water and, of course, from the creatures they saw around them.

The fighting skills and tactics of animals were much envied and copied.

Animals were a particularly strong source of inspiration as it was believed that animals had special, almost supernatural powers to help them survive the harsh environment and to be able to hunt prey and defend themselves successfully. The Shamans of ancient China were known as the wu and they were said to be able to communicate directly with animals and spirits and to be able to allow the spirit of an animal to enter their body and control their movements. When in this state they would make the movements and sounds of the animal and so may have inspired some fighting skills through this 'spirit possession'.

The Hundred Schools of Thought

The Chinese have long been inquisitive about themselves and how they fit into the world around them.

During the period from the 6th to the 2nd century BCE a wide range of thoughts and ideas were discussed and developed. This was known as the golden age of Chinese philosophy and produced what came to be known as the 'hundred schools of thought'. There weren't literally one hundred schools and of those that were developed during this period just two remain: Taoism and Confucianism. Taoism is concerned with how man fits into the natural laws and cycles of nature and Confucianism with how each individual fits into the social constructs and hierarchies of life. Taoists aim to be at one with the flow of the universe - the Tao where Confucianists aim more for a structured and harmonious society.

Buddhism found its way to China sometime around 60CE and it became the third of the trilogy of major Chinese philosophies that are still practised today. Indeed, it is estimated that by 500CE there were more than ten thousand Buddhist temples in China and many monks travelled to India to seek further knowledge or to bring back classic manuscripts. In the same vein, many Indian Buddhist monks travelled to China to teach.

The Beginning of Shaolin

One of these monks was the legendary Bodhidharma known to the Chinese as Da Mo. According to the legend in the year 527CE on his travels Bodhidharma went to the Buddhist temple of Shaolin in the Song Shan mountains where he found the meditating monks weak and sickly. Bodhidharma is said to have sat down facing a wall in meditation for nine years before emerging and teaching the monks a new set of exercises to build their strength and vigour. Bodhidharma stayed in the mountain temple all his life and died there. The exercises he

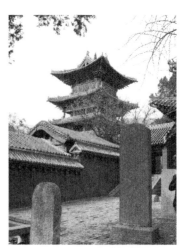
The Shaolin Monastery

taught were gradually developed and codified into fighting skills. Although it is clearly not true that kung fu started at Shaolin it is possible that it was at Shaolin where kung fu first became institutionalised and codified into set syllabuses.

Around 600CE some monks from Shaolin assisted the Qin King in a battle for which service he gave the Shaolin monastery some land and permitted them to train their own warriors. From then on martial arts training became a necessary part of the life of all Shaolin monks. For centuries to come Shaolin became a centre of Buddhist martial arts training. Within the temple walls of Shaolin, a wide range of kung fu styles were practiced and developed.

The Vastness of Wudang

Wudang became famous as the Taoist centre of martial arts in the same way that Shaolin was the Buddhist centre of the martial arts.

For centuries Wudang has been the spiritual and historical home of the internal martial arts. It was built on a grand scale with over two thousand temple buildings making it the world's largest centre of Taoism.

Wudang is not a single mountain but a range with twenty-seven peaks and covering an area of around two hundred square miles. The first Taoist temple was built on the Wudang mountain in the Tang dynasty around the 8th century. However, most of the temples were built during the Ming dynasty whose emperors wanted it built on such a grand scale. The temples housed as many as twenty thousand monks at any one time. Legend has it that after the three hundred thousand labourers had finished building the Forbidden City in Beijing the emperor ordered them to Wudang where they worked for the next ten years to create such a huge and beautiful monument to Taoism.

Within the temples of Wudang a wide range of skills were developed and practiced including many areas of medicine, spirituality, and other areas of human cultivation. Among the skills that were practiced and developed were the neijia – the internal martial styles of China. Legend has it that the Taoist monk Zhang Sanfeng created the art of t'ai chi chuan in Wudang and the area has been known as the home of the internal arts ever since.

The End of the Ming

Many kung fu styles were developed during the Ming dynasty (1368 - 1644) and it was during this time that Chinese martial arts were first introduced to Japan where they evolved into jujitsu and later judo.

The 1630s saw the beginning of the end for the Ming dynasty. The Manchus rebelled against the Ming dynasty and defeated the Ming army. The Chinese peasants who were over taxed and starving saw their chance and staged a revolt. The army who were themselves unpaid deserted Beijing without much of a fight. The last Ming emperor hanged himself from a tree in the imperial garden rather than face the ignominy of surrender. Over the next few years the Manchus gradually took over all of China to form the Qing dynasty.

During a large part of the Qing dynasty (1644 – 1911) martial arts training was forbidden as the ruling Manchus feared that the training of such skills may lead to a successful rebellion. Martial arts training continued but was driven underground in secret schools. It was during this period that the three major internal arts were developed: t'ai chi chuan, xingyiquan and baguazhang. Despite the precautions the 19th century saw a string of rebellions against the Manchus, each of which was put down but at enormous loss of life and resources. The Manchu central army was eventually destroyed and many local officials became warlords who used their private armies to rule independently in their provinces.

Civil War and The Shaolin Fire

From 1911, the Qing dynasty fell in a successful revolution led by Sun Yat Sen. The kung fu Masters were permitted to teach openly and the new Government encouraged them to open their schools to the public. Many kung fu books were written around this time. Sun was forced to turn power over to Yuan Shikai, the leader of the new army who had ambitions to be emperor. This was fiercely opposed even by his supporters and in 1916 he abdicated and died shortly after. This created a power vacuum in China which inevitably led to civil war. Two major sides evolved: the Kuomintang under Sun's protege Chiang Kai Shek and the Communist Party of China under Mao Zedong. In 1928 a battle took place close to the Shaolin temple which was set on fire.

The Shaolin fire was said to have raged for forty days and all the major temple building were destroyed and many priceless artefacts and training manuals were lost.

Around the same time as this Chiang Kai-Shek created the Nanjing Central Guoshu Institute. The aim of this institute was to preserve the martial arts of China. This was the first time that kung fu Masters broke their traditions of secrecy, sat down and shared knowledge with each other openly. The Institute held its first national martial arts competition which attracted four hundred of the best Masters in China. Later that same year a second tournament was held that attracted six hundred who were split into two categories: Shaolin and Wudang.

This seems to be the first time that the three arts of t'ai chi chuan, xingyiquan and baguazhang were officially recognised as Wudang arts. Unfortunately, the competitions were stopped after two Masters died and several more were seriously injured.

The ongoing civil war weakened China and allowed a successful Japanese occupation of the country from 1937. The two main civil war protagonists joined forces to fight the Japanese in the Sino-Japanese War which became part of the Second World War.

No Time to Train

During the Second World War and for a long time afterwards, survival was more important than martial training. The Japanese occupation was marked by horrific atrocities committed against the Chinese population. Their scorched earth policy also meant that even after the Japanese had surrendered in 1945 China was in the grip of severe famine.

Martial arts training became virtually impossible due to the famine, the Japanese atrocities and the still ongoing civil war. In 1949, the communist party emerged victorious and formed the People's Republic of China. Many of China's Masters left the homeland during those turbulent years and set up schools abroad, particularly in Hong Kong, Taiwan, the US and the UK. Initially they taught only Chinese immigrants but, eventually began to accept the local population into their ranks.

Standardised Kung Fu

In 1958, The Chinese Government decided to 'tame' the martial arts community and formed the All-China Wushu Association. The aim was to 'standardise' kung fu teaching in China. In reality, what happened was that virtually all of the vast combat knowledge that the arts represented was edited out of the forms and what was left was little more than a gymnastic display that could be taught to improve the people's health and be used as a showcase for the world stage. They combined the original kung fu forms with gymnastics, ballet and elements of Peking opera. The result does look amazing but it has almost no combat value.

There are two possible reasons for this purposeful blunting of the edge of kung fu. Almost certainly it was on the orders of the government to suppress the power of the Chinese boxers, the secret societies and the subversive nature of the family lineages. A plausible alternative is that it was done on purpose by the Masters themselves to prevent their skills and heritage from being exploited and given away by the government. Perhaps it was a bit of both but the end result was a sport called wushu that has traded awesome fighting functionality for flashy acrobatic movements.

Kung Fu's Darkest Hour

In 1966 Mao Zedong decided to enforce communism on the population by removing capitalist, traditional and cultural elements from society. This was perhaps the darkest time in China's long history and was known as the Cultural Revolution.

The traditional martial arts and philosophies of China were prime targets for persecution. Schools were closed down, Masters were imprisoned, temples were burned to the ground and training materials destroyed. Millions were persecuted and priceless knowledge relating to advanced kung fu training, human spiritual development, detailed medical texts and so on were burned or lost forever. This is possibly one of the greatest tragedies in human history. Nobody will ever know how much priceless knowledge is now gone forever.

The Cultural Revolution was the final blow for many of China's traditional schools and many of the Masters left China to settle down and teach elsewhere.

The Cultural Revolution dealt a near-fatal blow to the Chinese martial arts and the spiritual practices of Taoism which left both of them as mere shadows of their former selves.

The 70s Boom

In the 1970s Bruce Lee and David Carradine exploded onto our screens and the kung fu boom was born. Suddenly the Masters who had fled abroad and been teaching their fellow immigrants found themselves in demand from the population at large. Many of them held onto their traditions of secrecy and only taught their fellow Chinese. Others decided that their skills could be a benefit to all and so opened their schools to the occidentals as well. In the end, virtually all the Masters who could teach ended up taking 'foreign' students but the skills they taught them left out many of the critical power-generation practices.

The Digital Age

We now live in a digital age where any amount of information can be obtained with just a few clicks. It is now possible to research any kind of training and see videos and read articles. This is an opportunity that has never been available to martial artists before. In the past seeking out knowledge from other schools or teachers would have been seen as disloyal to one's own teacher and was much frowned upon but now it is becoming the norm. Unfortunately, the vast amount of information that is now available is often quite generic and lacks structure and detail. This makes it hard to do proper research on styles and the various skills they teach.

From the above brief history, we can chart the rise and fall of the Chinese martial arts. The heyday of the arts is said to have been in the latter stages of the Qing dynasty, around the end of the 19th century. During that time self-development through the martial arts, particularly the neijia (internal arts) became fashionable and flourished. People sought books and teachers who could expound secret training regimens to enable further personal growth.

The twentieth century saw the sad destruction of so much priceless knowledge, the loss of so many Masters and their schools and the gradual erosion of kung fu skills. Because of this, I think it is vital that the knowledge that is left is preserved for the benefit of a greater population and for the generations to come. This is why I have written this book and the books to come and have set up my online training site. They are an attempt to document the marvellous skills and principles that I have learned the hard way and make them available to a much wider audience. The technology of the twenty-first century can go some way to make up for the vast stupidities of the last century.

Chapter 5.
The Erosion of Kung Fu

In order to pass on a martial tradition to the next generation two things are required: time and stability. Time because as every teacher knows students come and students go. However, what is needed is at least one, preferably a few students who are willing to commit at least ten years to learning the full system and then be willing and able to pass it on to the next generation. More comprehensive traditions could take much longer than ten years to fully learn and understand. Although training manuals have been produced for many of the arts no book can ever replace time with the Master. Only the Master can help the student understand the intricacies of each movement, how it adapts to changing circumstances, how, when and where to apply force and so on.

It is only through physical contact, through sparring and hands on training that a martial art can be fully learned.

Many students were and still are unwilling or unable to put in the long-term training necessary to learn the complete art before becoming teachers themselves. Therefore, they only had a part of the art to teach and so many of the subtle intricacies of their art were lost. It is that final ten or twenty percent of the art, of course, that holds the most advanced skills and sought after treasures. Now we are left in many cases with the knowledge that certain skills were, perhaps, once possible but with nobody still alive to teach them to us.

Learning requires continuity

It is not just time but stability that is important in passing on a tradition. If you don't know where your next meal is coming from, if you are forced to defend your homestead, if your school is suddenly shut down or moved or your teacher disappears then no matter how motivated you are it becomes impossible for you to fully learn a system.

The twentieth century was a dark time for Chinese martial artists when for a very long period it was all but impossible to study long enough to fully comprehend an art. We lost at least one generation and when that happens the links to the old schools, the secrets that only the old Masters held were lost as they had nobody to pass them on to. Not just the old Masters but many of their training manuals were destroyed during the Cultural Revolution. From then on Chinese martial arts has become increasingly fragmented and we are now at the stage where you are probably more likely to find a good kung fu teacher outside China than you are within it.

The Lack of Experimentation

There is another reason why kung fu is dying out and this is the fault of the schools that teach it. A martial art, like any other form of human endeavour, can evolve only if its practitioners are willing to experiment. For most of kung fu's long history, its exponents would be constantly trying out new skills, different ways of training their mind and body, experimenting with power generation, tactics and so on. They had to be constantly innovative simply to survive. Without innovation, you had a set of skills that were carved in stone and if they weren't taught properly or any of them weren't passed on to the next generation then your art could only get weaker and weaker while the schools around that were innovative would get stronger and stronger.

In this modern era few traditional schools are prepared to experiment.

Most modern schools are too scared to deviate in any way from their set syllabus in case they 'get it wrong'. The sad truth is they are already getting it wrong. Often the skills they teach are ineffective and in some cases downright dangerous. They place themselves in positions that leave themselves wide open to attack, they have little idea about the primary importance of a strong structure and their movement skills are often unbalanced, barely coordinated and correspondingly weak.

Not all schools are like this - there are still good schools around but they are increasingly in the minority. And don't think it's just the Chinese martial artists who are unwilling to experiment. I have taught hundreds of different students from a wide variety of martial backgrounds and I can barely remember even one who has previously been to a school where experimentation was the norm. Yet without experimentation your art is dead or, at best, has reached its peak and is now going downhill. I was always taught not to take anything for granted but to experiment and find the best way.

These days there are so many books and videos and training courses and much of the information is contradictory. It is therefore up to you to experiment for yourself to discover which are the best methods for you. Don't take anyone else's word for it, no matter how famous or respected they appear to be. It may well be that methods that work for them won't work so well for you simply because they are not you. It may equally be that many teachers also can't get the moves to work in the way they'd like but they let their ego or their respect for the traditions of their school get in the way of admitting it. You are different in every way from everyone else so never be scared to experiment to find out what works best for you. This is true in every area of life, not just kung fu.

The Rise of Acrobatics

Acrobatic moves of all kinds are being increasingly taught in kung fu classes. Many schools are claiming that they have always been a part of the kung fu curriculum. I don't believe this is so and, if they have it has always been a minor part and didn't take up the same length of training time that many modern schools dedicate to it.

Acrobatic movements look great but are not conducive to realistic street combat. Firstly, they take your feet off the floor and this makes it impossible to develop a root which then makes it impossible to develop whole-body power. Secondly, while you are flying through the air you are very vulnerable to attack. Your body isn't stable in any direction so any kick or strike will injure you much worse than if you were. You are also unable to move out of the way of an attack if you are in mid-air or on your hands. Thirdly, a lot of energy is spent on leaping and rolling and flipping through the air. This is energy that isn't being spent on actual combat and the essence of good kung fu is total efficiency of movement.

There are good reasons for this emphasis on efficiency. In a real life and death situation it is quite likely that you would be attacked by several people at the same time. Certainly, that was the case in feudal China. To waste all your energy on leaping around and doing gymnastics while fighting the first person would leave you vulnerable to the others. Hence it was imperative that all your movement skills be as efficient as possible with nothing wasted so that you could take attackers down with minimal effort. Many people believe that flying kicks are an effective attack. Yes, they are effective but only if done against someone on horseback. That is what they were developed for as someone on horseback can't step out of the way of a flying kick.

The increasing usage of acrobatics in modern kung fu schools is partly down to its usage in modern wushu and partly down to the cinematic kung fu where the actors use acrobatics and wirework to add dramatic effect to their staged fights.

It should go without saying that it is increasingly difficult to perform acrobatic moves as you get older. They are fine, indeed fun, when you are in your teens, twenties, or thirties but beyond the age of forty they become increasingly difficult and risky. What do martial artists who only know these skills do when they get older? Many of them look to t'ai chi chuan for some gentle exercise that vaguely reminds them of some moves they used to do when they were young. Whereas if they trained their body properly using the principles of whole-body power and efficiency of movement they could still be fit, healthy and actively involved in the martial arts well into their old age.

Teaching the Confucian Way

The Chinese have always been extremely motivated to learn their kung fu. For many of them it was literally what would keep them and their family or clan alive. The more turbulent the age, the more the need for such skills existed. Even without that constant need for quality defensive skills, the Chinese were motivated from Confucian traditions of loyalty to one's family and one's school.

To not turn up for training would be to let yourself, your school and your family down. You literally became a part of the family of the school with your teacher taking the role of father and your fellow students your older or younger siblings.

In the Confucian manner of teaching the teacher would tell you what to do and you would do it, without question. Questioning your teacher was enormously disrespectful. More often than not teachers would show students how to do certain skills but not explain the principles that enabled them to be performed with effortless power. These principles were left to the student to work out if he could. It was one of the tests to see if the student was worthy enough to learn the higher levels of the art.

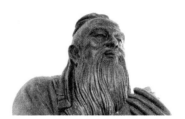

Confucius 551BC – 479BC

This is the way I was trained and it has taken me twenty odd years to work out the principles involved so that I am now able to perform these skills with the same effortless power as my own teachers.

Demonstrate, demand many repetitions but let students figure out how things work for themselves. This is the Confucian way.

Although I hugely appreciate the skills I gained I don't agree with the Confucian manner of teaching. It is inefficient and seems designed to keep the students hungry for knowledge as long as possible. Indeed, it is in large part to blame for the loss of good kung fu skill we have today.

It is not my way and I teach my students the principles of how to move with effortless power from the start. These principles are also to be found in this series of books for you to study and benefit from. However, reading them is one thing but incorporating them into your kung fu is quite another as many of them run contrary to the way you habitually think and move. So, if you read something that doesn't seem right don't take my word for it. Try it out for yourself and don't be afraid to experiment. The knowledge in this book works. It works for me and has worked on the hundreds of students I have taught and experimented with. But they are not you and neither am I.

Legends and Lineages

Most books on martial arts come complete with histories, lineages and legends of ancient warriors who were unbeatable in combat and humble in daily life. This book contains the bare minimum of such detail. Personally, I have always found them the least interesting part of a book. Lineages, no matter how well researched or how full of famous martial Masters can tell you next to nothing about how well any individual can fight and/or teach. Just because person X studied under Master Y that doesn't make them an equally good martial artist.

How long did they study under that Master? What exactly did they learn? What was their relationship to the Master - were they just one of hundreds of students or was there a much more personal, disciple type relationship involved? Lineages are often unable to answer these questions even about the direct students of a Master let alone about students several generations down. Would you want to learn how to fly an aircraft from someone who's only qualification is that his grandad used to fly and he handed down the knowledge?

It is more than likely that the full knowledge of a martial system won't have been passed on from every Master to even his highest student (let alone his many other students) as there may not have been time or indeed inclination to do so. Therefore, at every generation some of the content of the style may have been lost. Think about this logically. What are the chances that your teacher learned absolutely everything there was to learn from his teacher who, in turn, learned everything there was to learn from his own teacher and so on for generations back? I know that I haven't learned everything that my own teachers knew, not by a long way. However, I have filled in many of the gaps through research and experimentation. Few teachers do the same.

It is unfortunately true that many, once legendary kung fu styles are now just shadows of their former selves.

This isn't necessarily their fault but is partly down to Chinese history which made it all but impossible to study kung fu seriously for much of the twentieth century. On top of this is the extreme difficulty any good Master has in finding successors who are willing to put in the decades necessary to fully assimilate a complete art. After all, kung fu is one of the most difficult of skills to learn properly. It requires complete mastery of your body, mind and movements and the ability to adapt constantly to unpredictable circumstances which change at high speed.

Apart from the problems with lineages, every style has its own legendary fighters who did amazing things. After all these are the way in which the schools sell themselves to prospective students. However, few of these legendary deeds are in any way verifiable. So, legends and lineages have never been important to me. All that really matters is how much knowledge and skill a teacher really has and how much of that is he willing and able to pass on to you. Sometimes it is better to find a teacher who has only modest skill but is an excellent teacher than one who has incredible skill but is unwilling to pass it on or treats his students so badly that none will stay with him.

It surprises many people to learn that there is not now, nor ever has been, anything to stop anybody from setting up their own kung fu school and calling them self a Master. There are no governing bodies to register with, no officially recognised qualifications to take and nothing to stop you teaching what you want and calling yourself whatever you like.

In the past, any school that wanted to be taken seriously would have to prove themselves by showing their skills in combat. In this survival of the fittest environment the weaker schools would quickly die out and only the best would survive to pass on their training to the next generation. This is no longer the case. These days there is little or no risk that you will be challenged physically. Unfortunately, it is now the case that a great many so-called teachers or Masters are setting up schools and teaching rubbish to a public that doesn't know any better. After a while the public may realise that their teacher doesn't really know much and move elsewhere but if the teacher's marketing is good enough they will soon be replaced.

Traditional kung fu schools survived, and indeed differentiated themselves through legends and lineages. They would boast of famous martial heroes in their past, men of legend and tell how their training is the same as that of the legendary hero. They show you their school's family tree, their lineage to show a direct route from the heroes of old to their own training.

Both of my Masters maintained that lineages mean exactly nothing. It doesn't matter what the lineage is of the Master who taught you. All that matters is how much skill and power he has and how much of that he can impart to you. Yes, your teacher is important, in fact having a good teacher is more important than anything else but great teachers can come from little known lineages and very bad teachers may have a lineage full to the brim with famous, legendary Masters.

However, these legends and lineages are what kung fu has, what it's always had in place of qualifications and governing bodies. If you study almost any other discipline there will be qualifications to take and governing bodies to satisfy before you could practice or teach it. There has never been any organised network to standardise and promote the martial schools of China.

There have always been many secret societies that played a large part in the martial world of the Chinese fighters. During the centuries of imperial China, the saying was "The officials draw their power from the law; the people, from the secret societies." These societies often opposed the imperial government and are largely responsible for most of the rebellions and changes of dynasty that have occurred over many centuries. These societies became extremely powerful and they bound their members to them with secret oaths and initiation ceremonies in much the same way the Freemasons did. The Chinese societies functioned both as spiritual bodies and coordinating resistance to the government of the day. Although they have played an important role in Chinese society and were strongly tied to the martial schools they were never seen as governing bodies of kung fu.

So, the traditional schools try to persuade you that their lineages show an unbroken line of knowledge going back many generations. In truth, they can prove nothing of the kind. Particularly as we have seen that the twentieth century saw so much horror and bloodshed and so much destruction of the traditional schools and their prized knowledge.

The kung fu schools we have left should be judged on their own merits and not by the standards of previous generations.

Too many schools are surviving on past glories but without the skills to justify them. Much of what is taught today is a shadow of what once was. However, there are still gems to be found. Kung fu still has an awful lot to offer the world in terms of human development. So, let's take a look at that now.

Chapter 6.
Why Learn Kung Fu?

Good kung fu is not just for fighting but offers a path to follow to enable you to live a long, healthy and balanced life. Naturally few things are more detrimental to your health than having somebody try to hurt or kill you so the ability to defend yourself against attack is important. However, it is not as important now as it was when these arts were developed, unless you live in a particularly nasty neighbourhood. So, although it is unlikely that you will need to use your skills against a real assailant, it is very likely that you will need to fight the demons of stress, ill health and lack of balance in your life. Kung fu helps with all of these as well as the threat of physical assault.

Kung fu has so many benefits it's hard to know where to start. Perhaps I should start with what I feel my kung fu training has done for me.

Over the last thirty years I have found that my study of kung fu has helped me enormously in enabling me to accept myself and come to terms with the world around me. I have found that being more in control of my mind, body and emotions has helped me to gain the strength I needed to live life on my own terms without feeling the need to conform to this culture's increasingly shallow values.

Most people have so little connections within themselves that it's no wonder that they find it so hard to connect to anyone else or to the world around them. As a culture, we tend to live inside our minds, cut off from our bodies, indeed often actively hating our bodies which of course, leads to long term health issues in itself.

Our minds are at the mercy of our emotions which are in turn completely at the mercy of the slightest change in our environment.

Everything seems to be out of control, the body is a mass of habitual gestures, the emotions run riot at the slightest thing and the mind relentless goes round and round creating spirals of negative thought patterns that we cannot seem to control. I have found that my kung fu studies helped me to use my body more effectively and to become more stable emotionally thus giving me more control over my whole self. With this more integrated self I found that I was more effective at whatever I applied myself to as I was able to put more of myself into it. At the same time, I was less stressed when things didn't go smoothly. It has been a long process but I now enjoy trying to help people go through that same process in a much shorter time than it took me.

I find most people confused and bewildered by modern life. Nobody really feels as if they fit into our culture whereas if you look at more ancient cultures then everybody knew their position in society and so had more security and happiness than we, as a civilisation, do. Kung fu training helps by giving you such a strong sense of 'self' that no matter what circumstances you find yourself in you will have the physical and emotional resources to deal with it with relative ease.

Kung fu is a vast field of study. It has held my interest for over thirty years and I can't imagine ever growing bored of it.

In the study of kung fu there are always new skills to learn and higher levels to reach for all the while continuing to further develop the skills that you already know and love. Kung fu holds everything you could possibly want in an exercise system/martial art/self-development programme. It is the complete all-rounder in terms of developing your mind, body, energy, emotions, and spirit.

The highest levels of kung fu were developed by Buddhist and Taoist monks with the aim of protecting themselves from ill health and bandits while they were studying the physical and metaphysical aspects of the universe. They found that the training developed new levels of energy and focused power that they could bring to their meditations and that it complemented their spiritual aspirations perfectly. They developed principles and practices that enabled them to remain in a completely calm and meditative state even during hard physical exercise and the threat of personal injury or even death. All human beings naturally tense up when under pressure but the kung fu monks discovered ways to reverse this and defeat the injurious effects of stress. This gave them better physical and mental health as well as superior fighting skills. Some of these skills are covered in my book 'Stress Proof Your Body'.

Here are just a few of the myriad benefits of kung fu.

Balanced training

The first priority for people new to kung fu is to bring their body back into balance. Most people are carrying way too much tension particularly in their shoulders and hips. These areas becoming chronically tight and lead to long term joint problems. Long periods of time spent sitting down weaken the leg and back muscles. Kung fu training strengthens the legs and core muscles and opens up the hips and shoulders to bring your body back into balance.

Chinese martial arts (and particularly Taoist and Buddhist ones) focus on achieving balance not aggression. You aim to achieve balance within yourself, in your movements, your emotions, your breathing and so on. When you have balance inside yourself then it is much easier to find balance in the environment and with the people around you. You learn to generate power that flows through your whole body rather than over exerting any particular part. You also strive to seek balance with your opponent, learn to merge with his attacks, learn to become sensitive to his movements so that you can react instantly and with fluid power so that you are never caught off guard or off balance.

Kung fu works the body, mind, and breath together to restore equilibrium to the practitioner. This helps them maintain good health and fitness throughout their life.

I am firmly of the belief that the human body is capable of healing from any illness or injury providing that it is kept in a state of balance. It is when the body is kept out of balance by lack of exercise, poor dietary choices and high levels of physical tension that that we become unable to heal naturally. I try to be the embodiment of this. I am now in my early fifties yet I have all my own teeth and hair, have no need for glasses, take no medication at all for anything and am in excellent health. I currently teach seven classes a week and constantly have to prove to people half my age or younger that I am fitter and healthier than they are.

I can manage this because kung fu not only offers comprehensive physical training but also trains the other aspects of the human organism. Westerners are only now starting to realise the importance of mindfulness, of awareness training, of working with the breath and so on. Yet these have been a focus of training in China for thousands of years. The world of kung fu takes from all of these and uses them to develop the individual in many and sometimes extraordinary ways.

Comprehensive Skills

Kung fu is not a single martial art like judo is. There are hundreds of different kung fu styles. Some of these styles are similar but there are also vast differences to be found between most of them and even many differences between the teachings of one school and another even of the same style.

As there is such an enormous range of kung fu skills nobody can master them all in one lifetime. Many martial arts and kung fu styles tend to focus on certain aspects of training and combat such as kicking skills or grappling.

What kind of skills does a good kung fu school offer? Each school will offer at least some of the following:

1. General body conditioning.
2. Specific conditioning to develop particular skills.

3. Striking and kicking skills of various levels of advancement.

4. Grappling skills (locks, holds and throws).

5. Pressure point knowledge.

6. Knowledge of biomechanical alignments to make each movement efficient and powerful.

7. Forms - preferably functional rather than just decorative.

8. Weapons training.

9. Sparring practices.

10. Developing the body from the inside e.g. qigong and other breathing and slow-motion efficiency drills.

11. Developing the mind through different types of meditation.

12. A coherent philosophy that underpins everything that's taught.

Any one of the above could take many decades to fully master so don't expect that your school will be able to teach all of these to a high level. For example, there are over a hundred pressure points and each one requires different amounts of pressure and to be attacked from the right angle. Some of them won't work at all unless a joint is held in a certain way and some people seem relatively immune to any and all of them. It's a lot to learn. Similarly, there are many weapons and most Masters will only be proficient at a handful of them.

Over a hundred different weapons have been used by Chinese martial artists over the centuries.

The martial art elements that are important to you may not be so important to someone else so if you're looking for a good martial arts school take the above list and put them in your order of preference then go and talk to the local instructors and their senior students to see how well they could fit in with your needs and wishes.

Any martial art that ticks all the boxes above could be described as a complete martial art. To study a complete martial art means you learn to deal with a huge range of different attack/defence scenarios. You become comfortable at defending yourself from all ranges and from all directions. You should know how to deal with long, medium and short-range weapons and be able to use them yourself. You should also understand how different martial arts develop power and be able to deal with that. And all of these things must be done while your mind and body remain calm and free of tension.

The study of a complete martial art takes a very long time - usually the whole of your life

It takes a long time but it is time that is spent on developing yourself in a myriad of ways. You start to understand the forces that can act upon you and the most efficient ways for you to balance and control those forces. You develop a sense of your environment and martial tactics, you gain speed and decisiveness of thought and you also learn the most important lesson of all - that the only opponent in life you need to deal with is yourself.

If you are attacked in the street your opponent is giving you a set of tactics and forces to deal with. Will the various parts of yourself come together to deal with that scenario successfully, or won't they? Study enough, train enough and they will.

Having spent the last thirty years studying a complete martial art that ticks all the above boxes I have seen many students come from a wide variety of martial arts schools that seem to be lacking in so many fundamental areas.

Their movements lack any coordinated power, they have been taught to place themselves in vulnerable positions such as one hand being kept on the back hip where it is of little use, they try to use dangerous movements that lead them wide open to simple counters and so on.

These bad practices seem to be more prevalent now than they were even a few years ago. I teach a well-formed structure that uses the whole body to control and manipulate the space all around you with balanced power. I emphasise how important it is not to focus all your attention on the one attacker but to stay alive to the whole situation around you.

There is so much more to martial arts training than most people, even experienced martial artists, realise. We are fortunate in this day and age to have access to books, DVDs and YouTube videos of other styles and practitioners and to be able to use these to widen our own knowledge base and see where our weaknesses lie.

Adaptability

Kung fu teaches you to become highly adaptable. You learn to be sensitive to what is going on around you and then to adapt your tactics and skills to match. People do wild and desperate things in combat and you must be prepared mentally and physically for pretty much anything.

In kung fu, if something you try doesn't work immediately, try something else.

If you're trying to apply an armlock and the person isn't responding to it don't try going harder and harder. That would mean you're just pitting your strength against theirs. You end up wasting your energy and tying yourself up with tension. This isn't the kung fu way. I always tell students that no movement they do on anyone should take more than fifty percent of their strength. As they become more advanced that percentage should go down. I never use more than ten to twenty percent on my students but it's more than enough to put them down or in considerable pain. If you need more than fifty percent in any move then change the move into something similar. If you're trying to do a circular arm lock then let go of the arm and turn it into a circular strike instead. The move is the same it's just the way you apply it changes.

It is the people who are flexible in their approach to life who thrive where those who are stuck in their ways become miserable and struggle to survive. Kung fu teaches you to stay in the moment and adapt to whatever comes your way with all of your mind, body and heart.

Everybody on the earth is unique as is every situation in which you find yourself. There is no one technique or skill that will work every time - if there was you wouldn't need to learn anything else. What is important is not individual techniques but movements that are able to adapt to different techniques instantly as required. It is this essential ability to adapt each movement you have that is missing from most modern martial arts forms.

A strong and healthy structure

A major benefit that differentiates kung fu training from Western sports or fitness training is the emphasis on both internal and external training. Apart from the usual methods of physical training, strength, flexibility, speed and so on, there is a much greater emphasis on the training of the mind, the mental connections between brain and body, precise coordination between parts of the body, sensitivity training and a much wider range of movements in the joints than you will find in any Western exercise system. These are of enormous benefit to the health of the practitioner and enable him or her to maintain a high degree of health and fitness well into old age.

Kung fu develops a certain type of body that differs from usual fitness training

Kung fu training develops a body that doesn't hold on to unnecessary tension, one where every part of the body supports all other parts and everything is moving with the ultimate efficiency, aligned with gravity and using the bigger muscles of the lower body more than the smaller muscles of the upper body. It also develops calmness of mind and spirit as what happens in the mind is reflected in the body and vice versa. You learn to change instantly from soft, flowing moves to hard, fast and powerful ones where needed.

Kung fu offers a point to physical exercise.

It's infinitely more rewarding and interesting than going to any gym, which I find mind-numbingly tedious. You know that you are learning skills that have been developed over hundreds, even thousands of years and tested endlessly under real life or death situations. If these skills didn't work or were detrimental to your health they wouldn't have lasted so long. Having said that there are a number of practices that are bad for your health that you find in some martial arts schools, but not in the good kung fu schools.

To get these benefits for yourself you need to find a good kung fu school. These aren't easy to find so let the next chapter help you on your quest.

Chapter 7.
Finding a Good School

Now that I've whetted your appetite I hope that you will take up the challenge and want to learn kung fu yourself. After all, why else would you buy this book? Unfortunately, you cannot learn kung fu from this or any other book, online training site or video. In this volume, I aim to give you an excellent introduction to kung fu. By the end of it you will know several exercises and skills and how you can use them for real. However, this is in no way a substitute for real study with a good Master.

Only a good Master can see what you are doing wrong and correct you. Only in a class environment do you have access to a range of different people to try your skills on. The best I can hope to do here is inspire you to find a good teacher and give you some usable skills to make your first few sessions easier. Kung fu is all about person to person contact so it's something you need to feel and experience first-hand with a genuine Master and by working with a range of students in a class environment.

Having the right teacher is far more important than learning the right style.

Make no mistake it is the teacher him or herself who will make the most difference to your training. Here are a few pointers in finding the right teacher and the right school for you.

It is often said that learning a martial art is like climbing a mountain. All books and DVDs can do is give you a map of the initial terrain you will cover and some vague paths that may be able to take you part of the way up. What is really required is a teacher who is willing and able to walk with you up the path, pushing you ahead of him where possible and guiding you over the rough spots that you will face. Without a teacher, it is easy to go off the path and end up confused and alone. In fact, without a good teacher it is impossible to go more than a part of the way up anyway as no book, article or video will really reveal the inner secrets of any system. Indeed, in this book I can merely scratch at the surface of just the first fundamental elements of the system I have studied for over thirty years. The subsequent books will reveal more of the system but again can only hint at certain skills as describing them fully isn't possible in a book. Also, there are many levels of complexity beyond these skills and these can't be shared in a book but can only be passed on physically to students.

The first thing to understand is that, when it comes to learning kung fu, it is more about the teacher than the style. You may have your heart set on learning bagua, or hung gar or wing chun or whatever style but there may not be a school teaching that style in your area so you have to choose between the schools that are available to you. If you live in a city you probably have a good choice. If you're more rural then your choice may be very limited indeed. You should visit the schools available to you, see if you can get a free intro lesson and if possible talk to the teacher and more senior students to get a feel for what they're offering. After all, if you're going to be studying at this school these will be your role models so are they the kind of people with the kind of skills you're looking for?

Traditional martial arts vs combat sports

It is important at the outset for you to decide if you want to learn a combat sport that is involved in competition or a traditional martial art. There are advantages and disadvantages to both.

Most kung fu schools are traditional schools and are focused on real life combat and self-development, not training in a competitive sport. Combat sports are fun to learn but do have more limitations than traditional arts in that the techniques you will learn are more geared towards success in competition. On the plus side, their use of protective equipment and combat rules means they can spar with more power and ferocity than you would find in most traditional schools, many of whom don't spar at all. I am a traditional arts man and always have been but only as long as the arts are realistic and are trained effectively. When a traditional art is trained properly I, personally, believe it to be better than a combat sport.

In any combat sport, the environment is known – it's an empty ring or cage, the opponent is known and he will have trained the same way you have so you already know what he can or can't do. You both have to follow the same rules and wear the same clothing. In real-life violent encounters, the environment is unfamiliar and changing all the time. There are no rules to fall foul of and no referee to step in to prevent serious injury. All combat sports focus on one man against one man and this makes it utterly different to real street conflict where the chances are you will face many opponents at the same time. Therefore, the way you fight must be different than if you were fighting one man in a ring with rules and a referee. Traditional schools teach people different tactics than you will have seen in any combat sport environment. In real life it can be dangerous, even fatal to focus all your attention on one man. You must be constantly moving and alive to everything that is going on around you. There are tactics and methods that will enable you to do this but you won't find them in any combat sport.

Traditional martial arts are also more focused on the development of your mind and body through the learning of what were once battlefield skills. The skills I teach use the whole body for attack and defence and are used to defend the individual from multiple attackers. The training also focuses on remaining calm inside while under pressure from outside. The aggression that is encouraged and displayed during most martial arts competitions is alien to such training. Our focus is on staying calm and being unaffected by your attacker's aggressive attitude.

Belts and gradings

When people think of martial arts one of the commonest symbols is that of a black belt. The use of coloured belt rankings is now ubiquitous but it is a fairly recent phenomenon. The whole idea of giving coloured belts depending on one's rank and knowledge started with the Japanese art of Judo in the mid-1930s and it was so simple and effective that it rapidly spread. Most Japanese, Okinawan and Korean martial arts soon adopted the system. Most traditional kung fu schools don't use any coloured belt or sash system although gradually more and more are now realising its benefits.

I have been teaching since 2003 and finally adopted the coloured belt system in 2015. I find it extremely useful when teaching a complicated physical art form to be able to know at a glance exactly what any student knows and what they still need to learn. Before I adopted the system, it was impossible to keep track of which student had learned what skill and to what level. So, students were progressing to fairly advanced skills yet still missing some fundamental knowledge.

Unfortunately, many schools simply use belt rankings as an extra income for the school and dish them out every couple of months or so. This diminishes the value of the belt and leads to 'black belt factories' that can guarantee a black belt within a year or some other such laughable timescale. Each of the sash colours that I grade on requires a set of skills to be mastered and pressure tested before I'm happy enough to award the sash and certificate. When you have to work hard to earn something you have much greater respect for it.

What to look for in a teacher

Finding a good teacher is a matter of luck as well as judgement. Unfortunately, the chances of you living close to a teacher who is willing and able to teach you all you need to know isn't high which is the one of the reasons why I wrote this book. There are a lot of people who claim to teach kung fu but many have few usable skills and waste a lot of their student's time doing basic conditioning exercises in class that could and should be done at home.

As I mentioned before there is nothing to stop anybody calling themselves a kung fu teacher and setting up their own school. There are no regulations, no recognised qualifications and no laws against it. Obviously, this has led to thousands of people doing just that with minimal or no training at all and just hoping to make some money and have a huge boost to their ego at the same time. I will teach you how to spot these 'kung fu cowboys' shortly.

On the whole, the good teachers who are out there are humble. They often don't bother with fancy uniforms or titles. Their movement skills may not look flashy but they are highly effective and extremely powerful. They don't need posh looking premises nor do they try to tie students into long contracts. Some may be strict disciplinarians where others, such as myself, are more laid back in their approach and prefer to instil self-discipline in their students.

Below are a few of the things that should start ringing alarm bells when looking for a good school and a suitable teacher and hopefully should cause you to avoid the school. The 'cardinal sins' include:

- Any school that teaches kung fu alongside other martial arts or combat sports such as kickboxing, jujitsu etc. No genuine kung fu Master would be seen dead teaching or promoting any art other than his own. If they have to teach kickboxing alongside kung fu it only proves how bad their kung fu must be!

- An egocentric or bullying approach towards the students. This can also come from the senior students who are encouraged to exert their authority. Senior students should be there to mentor you and help you as the teacher when he isn't around. After all, the teacher can't be everywhere, particularly in large classes. But avoid like the plague any teacher or senior student who belittles you or doesn't take your training seriously.

- Overemphasis on basic conditioning exercises. Some schools spend 75% of their class time or more on basic drills like running, skipping and press-ups. These things are important and will get you fit, to a point but you aren't learning martial arts and that is what you are paying for. If a class is spending a lot of time on these 'filler' activities it usually means the instructor doesn't have many skills to teach and wants to fill class time with other stuff. You can run around and do press-ups at home. Class time should be used to do things you can't do at home. Specifically, it should be used firstly to learn new skills and further develop old ones and, secondly to give you the opportunity to practice your skills with a range of partners.

- An insistence to tie students into a contract. Some of these contracts are up to three years and if you don't pay they refer it to a debt collection agency. If it is a good school offering quality tuition then students will want to stay and shouldn't feel financially forced into doing so.

- A teacher who won't answer questions. If you ask a teacher a relevant question, particularly one such as why you do a movement a certain way he should be able to answer you and demonstrate the reason why. If he refuses to answer, discourages questions or hides behind answers like 'that is how we do things in this style' then he doesn't understand his own style fully and may well be teaching you stuff by rote that may well not work for real.

- A school that sticks rigidly to teaching the same forms in exactly the same way every time to everyone. As I mentioned earlier on in this book any form that isn't adaptable is next to useless and won't serve you in combat. We are all different and react differently to every technique thrown at us. Every situation is different so your forms must be able to change quickly and smoothly to allow for the ever-changing winds of combat. Teachers who teach their forms the same way to everyone have either been taught that way themselves in which case the true meanings and skills of their forms were lost generations ago or are too lazy to teach them properly.

- A school that doesn't teach you the real combat skills of your forms and how to adapt them if the opponent doesn't react the way you'd like. It's also important to learn how to use them against non-compliant partners.

Real tuition from an experienced teacher is by far the best way of learning kung fu so it is worth spending some time checking out the schools in your local area to find out which one would be best for you. Each school is different, it has its own methods of training, its own ethos and focuses of different aspects of the kung fu 'experience'. To find the school that suits your needs best you really need to visit each one and talk to the teacher and the senior students to get a feel if this is a school you want to be associated with long term. Go along to a few lessons to get a feel for the way they are run and how you will progress. Don't rely just on websites as often schools with great looking sites may be poorly run or vice versa.

The challenges of teaching

I can tell you from experience that teaching kung fu is, in many ways, more difficult than teaching in a school or even teaching a martial art like karate which is often taught in quite a regimented style with a set syllabus and everything is named and taught in the same way every time. This makes it both easier to teach and easier to learn. As a kung fu teacher you have trained and developed a wide range of skills and these skills are fluid and constantly adaptable. You know, or should know, the main principles that make them work. Now you have a huge job of trying to present all this material to your students in a way that makes sense and keeps them interested. Usually in the smaller kung fu schools there is little in the way of a set syllabus to follow, you may have to develop your own. This means breaking down everything you know into simple steps and codifying them. It often means trying to remember how you first learned it a decade or more ago.

You need to be able to explain complicated concepts simply and demonstrate them effectively. You need to be adaptable enough to change the way you teach to meet the needs of the student in front of you whether they be a seven-year-old girl or a six foot plus ex-soldier. Every session needs to be planned and you must be prepared to abandon the plan at a moment's notice if the group in front of you is different than you expected. I've lost count of the times I've had to rethink an entire lesson plan while warming up the class.

I tell you all this so that you are aware of the pressures on the instructor in front of you. You cannot judge a class effectively from just one lesson – any instructor can have an off day. However, if you spot any of the cardinal sins that I mentioned above even in the first session I'd recommend you don't go back for a second one.

Kung fu titles

In order to attract students many Western teachers are giving themselves increasingly high-sounding titles. First it was Master, then Grandmaster now the ridiculous term Great Grandmaster is being used by some. Some teachers even call themselves Doctor or Professor despite having no accredited qualifications to merit those titles.

Most kung fu titles are meaningless as there is nothing to stop anyone giving themselves any title they like. Traditional Chinese martial arts were based on Confucian values of duty to one's family and one's school. When you were admitted to a school they became your second family. Your teacher became your father and your fellow students were your brothers and sisters. You would stay with the same teacher for many years until he was satisfied that your skill level was high enough for you to teach your own class within the school without bringing down the standards of the school. Even then you'd teach under the watchful eye of your teacher. The traditional term Sifu means teacher/father so it shows a deeper relationship than a school teacher has to his students. The teacher's teacher is called a different name which varies according to which part of China the school originates from. In English, we sometimes use the term Master. So, to become a Master you must have taught students who are now teachers themselves. When there is more than one Master in a school then the senior one and head of the school can be called Grandmaster. This is only to distinguish the most senior Master from the other Masters. These titles aren't self-appointed but are earned through a lifetime of training and dedication to one school and one art.

Many genuine Masters are humble men who don't use their titles and are happy to be referred to as Sifu, Teacher or even just by their name.

Many Masters are now ashamed of their titles as they have been cheapened and denigrated by the many rogues who claim fancy titles but offer no real skill or knowledge.

A formal title or lack of one in a teacher may mean nothing. There seems to be an inverse relationship these days between the fanciness of the title and the actual amount of knowledge and skill a teacher has. So, when looking for a good teacher ignore the titles and ranks and look for the skill i.e. how effortlessly and powerfully can he apply his techniques and movements and how well can he adapt them to the changing winds of combat.

The true kung fu Master

"Those who know do not speak. Those who speak do not know."

Over the last thirty years I have been fortunate enough to meet several genuine Masters of kung fu. Some I have studied with and others I just know. I have also met several who give themselves fancy titles but don't really have the 'juice' of kung fu. The real Masters are all very much individuals yet they all have certain traits that the pretenders lack.

Individuality

Kung fu Masters are singular men. They have walked a long road that few others have had the tenacity to walk. They have invested thousands of hours in training themselves and will have sacrificed much to do so.

They tend to have little or no interest in the things that others spend (waste) their time and money on: fashion, soap operas, computer games, gossip and so on. They are completely unmoved by fads and bandwagons. Kung fu Masters live their life their own way on their own terms.

Kung fu teaches you to become rooted. This is much more than just a physical process. The normal man or woman has little in the way of physical or emotional rooting. They are like a cork bobbing in a big ocean. As such they are at the mercy of wind and waves and follow whichever wind is strongest at the time. The kung fu Master is like a mighty vessel. It is on a course and neither storms nor the strongest ocean currents can divert it from its destination. This single-mindedness means that the Masters I have had the privilege of knowing have enormous levels of self-discipline. They are decisive about things that matter but couldn't care less about the trivialities of life that others spend their lives on. As such they tend to have few friends but value the ones they have.

Presence

The Masters I have known have extraordinary presence and charisma. Years of mental and physical focus have made every movement efficient and powerful. When they walk into a room they own the room and this is noticeable by others. When they look at you, their gaze can have such intensity that you feel they are looking into your very soul. They can switch this power on and off at will. Others who haven't studied kung fu can have a similar effect but without the innate power that kung fu brings.

Marilyn Monroe for instance could do much the same thing. On one occasion, she travelled on a train and sat in a normal carriage and was completely unrecognised. She was just plain old Norma Jean. Then she arrived at the station, decided to make an entrance, and simply struck a pose and instantly was surrounded by people who suddenly recognised her as Marilyn Monroe.

Another aspect of presence is internal connections. Kung fu Masters have learned to bring every part of themselves into everything they do. The arms and legs work together in perfect union with the head and torso. This is coordinated with the breathing and the mind and spirit are fully focused on what they are doing. It is this internal connection that is the mark of a true Master. Most normal people are completely disconnected. The arms and legs are uncoordinated, the body is unbalanced, the breathing is ragged and the mind is somewhere else entirely. This is why they don't have any real presence.

Kung fu Masters do not react to the world in the same fearful way that normal people do.

Genuine Masters have learned the hard way to be relaxed when in danger. Any excess tension that comes from fear will only get in the way of efficient and powerful movement. This self-control comes from mental focus and breath control along with countless hours facing opponents in mock combat. This skill set gives them the complete confidence in themselves and their skills. They know themselves inside out. They have met and come to terms with any limitations or weaknesses. They have no pretences and they no longer have anything left to prove to anyone much less themselves.

Most people think they know themselves but they are too disconnected from themselves and the world around them to really understand why they react in the ways that they do. Hence, they constantly feel the need to prove themselves to others in the vain hope that others will take their surface actions at face value and not see the turmoil and self-doubts within.

It is this combination of relaxed, yet alert manner, internal connection, physical control and mental focus that gives some people such amazing presence and makes them stand out from the crowd.

Humility

The Masters I have known have extraordinary skills yet they remain humble. They never brag or show off what they can do but keep their skills hidden from others. Their skill is their sword – they believe it should never be taken out and shown to others but should be kept sheathed until it is really needed. People only brag or show off when they feel they have something to prove. It is a sure sign of insecurity and weakness.

Real Masters know what they can do and that is enough. There is no need to have to prove it to others.

Once you start bragging about your skills then people want to see a demonstration. Particularly when it comes to extraordinary skills people say they won't believe it unless they see it and feel it. So, you feel obliged to demonstrate it and wow them. But then somebody else wants a demonstration, should you have to demonstrate it to them as well? There are seven and half billion people in this world so that could be an awful lot of demonstrating. The Master cuts out all this hassle by keeping his skills to himself.

Extraordinary Power

Finally, of course, the true Master has extraordinary physical power. This power is completely unrelated to his physical size. I have known and trained with Masters who were little more than five feet tall and weighed not much more than one hundred pounds but whose power had to be seen and felt to be believed. This awesome power didn't come from large muscles – almost none of the real Masters I know are what you'd call buff. Real power comes from internal connections, making every part of your body move together as one large muscle, connected by a focused mind and powered by a strong breath. This only comes from thousands of hours of practice.

There are many men out there who call themselves Master. Do they have the presence, the humility, the self-control and extraordinary power of a true Master or are they just pretending?

If you too want to walk with absolute power and confidence and to live your life completely on your own terms then practice today, practice tomorrow and keep practising. Make your body a worthwhile expression of your life and learn to become a realised person at one with yourself, your fellow man and the world around you. Read on to find out how.

PART 2 - TRAINING

Chapter 8.
The Basics of Training

Kung fu training revolves around developing the 'kung fu body'. That is a body that is free of unnecessary tension, flexible, able to withstand severe forces and able to generate great power with effortless ease. Moreover, it is a body that will last the whole of your life, it won't start falling apart when you are only in your forties, or even earlier. To gain the kung fu body you need to develop flexibility and connected strength. Everyone knows that flexibility is about how flexible your joints are i.e. how far you can stretch. Connected strength may be new to you. With connected strength, the focus isn't on the strength of specific muscles but how much force can be applied through many muscles groups in the body working precisely together. But before we get into the specifics we need to look at a few general points of kung fu training.

Generic vs Specific Training

Generic training involves general training for the body such as stretching exercises, push ups, leg strengthening exercises and so on. These are important, particularly early on in training to ensure you have a basic level of strength and flexibility. However, many schools overemphasize such generic conditioning in their classes and use them to fill time. This is a sure sign that they don't have many genuine skills to teach.

Most people today live sedentary lives. We no longer go on long walks to collect food, work in the fields or wash our clothes by hand. We spend around 90% or more of our days sitting down and this plays havoc with our bones, joints and muscles. Our legs become weak from lack of use. Our hips tighten as the main joints aren't being moved. Our backs and core muscles also weaken and become distorted from the unusual positions they sink into every day in our chairs. Our shoulders tighten as we do so many small movements with the hands and arms and the shoulders tighten up to hold the arms in unusual positions to work at a keyboard or move a steering wheel. As a result of these imbalances we are a mess. We also pay almost no attention at all to our body or how we are using it unless it starts to hurt. Even then we try to shut it up with painkilling drugs. Then we wonder why we are so stressed and ill.

If this is you then you need to start with some generic training to increase your stamina, flexibility and leg strength in particular. Then you can work on your upper body strength as well but don't overdo it. Our culture praises upper body strength over lower body strength. The fitness magazines are full of articles of how to get the six pack abs and the bulging biceps but these shouldn't be a priority.

In kung fu we develop the body as a triangle with the power at the base and less strength needed at the top. This is the way our bodies have evolved to work naturally.

Specific training is training to attain and develop specific skills such as striking skills, kicks, connected circular movements, form work and so on. When you have attained a reasonable level of generic fitness at least half of your training time should be spent on specific training skills. Class work should certainly be spent more on specific training rather than generic training which the practitioner can and should do at home in their own time. In this section, we will cover first some generic training exercises and then move onto specific training.

Naming techniques

Before we continue I want to talk briefly about the practice of naming exercises and specific movement skills. Each martial arts style will undoubtedly have its own names for specific exercises and movements. These may well be the same exercises and movements that are taught in other arts but have different names. This doesn't mean that one school is right and all the others are wrong but that they developed in different times and places and so gave their exercises and movements differing names.

Some martial arts, particularly the Japanese ones, have names for everything. Each skill has a distinct name which should be learned along with the skill. This makes teaching easy as everything has a name and is performed the same way every time so it is easy to check if it is done 'correctly'. This is, however, limiting.

If every skill has a name and is always performed the same way then it becomes set in stone and is no longer adaptable.

As I mentioned in the previous section any skill that is no longer adaptable to the constantly changing circumstances of combat is of limited use. In the system I teach there are very few names. Stances and circular movements with the arms have names but there aren't even names for many of the forms I teach. Specific techniques don't have names apart from a few that the students have given their own names to such as the seatbelt technique or the chawa punch kick. Many movements can look identical to each other yet have different applications depending on how they are used so giving everything specific names is impossible.

Alsokung fu has a far greater range of techniques and movements than you'd find in the combined karate and jujitsu syllabuses. This means finding individual names for them would be a daunting task. If our movements don't have specific names then how are they taught and remembered? Simply as part of forms or as movements that are similar to other movements in forms.

Learning a martial art is like learning a new language. You don't start by learning all the words beginning with A before moving onto words beginning with B. You learn by learning simple words then put them together into sentences and then paragraphs etc. You learn by telling stories. A form is like a story made up of several words. The opponent tells the other side of the story. Hidden within the form are the answers to any statement or question the opponent may make within the story. Each movement must be practiced both on its own and within the context of the form. To try to give each movement a name would be harder than trying to learn the written language of China itself which has tens of thousands of pictograms, each one representing a word or idea.

The Kung Fu Body

Back to the kung fu body. In order to develop it certain types of training are required:

Flexibility Training

This includes various stretching exercises to open the joints and stretch the muscles, tendons and other soft tissues. These essential exercises increase your mobility and enable your body to withstand the forces that act upon it. Flexible joints enable you to move into positions that others find difficult. They also help slow down the effects of ageing. A flexible body is one that does not allow a build-up of tension to prevent full freedom of movement. Flexibility prevents injuries and allows your posture to be properly aligned. In short, flexibility feels great and is the cornerstone of most Eastern exercise systems and with good reason.

Static Power Training

This means learning to stand still in various positions and allowing your body to relax into that position. While holding these positions you don't allow your physical structure to collapse at all yet you aim to release any unneeded tension. Gradually this allows each part of your body to add to the support of the whole. It develops your physical structure so that your body becomes extremely stable in fixed positions. Static power training is the most vital element of developing effortless, whole body power and is a crucial part of most respected kung fu styles. It delivers great health benefits as well as adding to your martial power.

Movement Drills

These train you to move your body as a whole rather than using just, say, the arms and shoulders. It's crucial that you learn to use your legs and waist in all your movements. You learn to feel the connections between all the body parts and use them to spread the movement and impact forces through all your muscles rather than just a few. This can be done with any of the kung fu movements or forms. It is best to select something simple to start with and do it with full focus ensuring that all movements are powered by the legs and directed by the centre and the power flows through relaxed arms. Gradually you learn to use your body in a relaxed, powerful, and very efficient way. You focus on performing the movements slowly to ensure that all the parts of yourself are working together and no part is rushing ahead.

Breath Training

This teaches you to use your breathing to maintain your physical energy and to release and prevent internal blockages. Your breath will help you to release unneeded tension and direct power to where it's needed. Breathing brings energy into the body and supports you from the inside. Without good breathing practices, a kung fu body is simply not possible.

Mind Training

Your mind controls your body so the more focused your mind becomes then the more powerfully it can control your movements and other physical functions. There becomes no lag between thought and action. Your mind inhabits your body and your movements mirror your thoughts. Your mind needs to become more disciplined so that it can remain focused on the task at hand. Instead of allowing it to be at the whim of the ego - forever moving from one topic or worry to the next, you must learn to train it to stay still in the here and now. This is one of the most empowering things you can do with your time.

These are the main areas but there are others such as specific conditioning exercises, balance training, sensitivity training and so on. Each of these building blocks needs to be trained regularly so that, when you need it, you are able to bring all that you are into everything you do.

The exercises in this book cannot cover all this training. It can only take you so far. It will not cover breath or mind training for example although these will be covered in later books. Also, there is information about both in my first book 'Stress Proof Your

Body' along with more information about how to develop a strong yet relaxed structure, among much else.

How to train

Here are a few points that will help you get the most out of your personal training time.

Dedicated, Mindful Practice

Kung fu means attainment through practice. Lots of practice. It cannot be gained just from reading books or articles or from watching videos although these can guide you on your way. Kung fu skill is gained and measured only through many thousands of repetitions of basic movements and training in specific exercises. These repetitions gradually change your body, making it feel stronger and lighter. They also change the way you move and express yourself. You gain new and more efficient movement habits. You learn to use your whole body powered by your breath and controlled by a more focused mind but, only if you practice regularly and conscientiously.

Much of the exercise we do in modern times is mindless.

We listen to iPods while jogging or watch TV screens when in the gym. Anything to take our minds outside of our body so that we can help the time go faster. Kung fu should never be mindless. It is important to keep your mind on your practice. You will find that there are a lot of things to focus on such as how you are breathing or feeling the connections between different parts of your body. By learning to keep your mind inside your body when you move you make all your movement skills more efficient. Your reflexes speed up and you gain an amazing level of balance and coordination. Kung fu is as much about training the mind as it is the body so try not to distract your mind but learn to train it so that you gain a razor-sharp focus.

Keep to the core skills

Please be aware when using this book not to get caught up in the excitement of continually learning new skills.

Every skill is only as strong and useful as the number of hours you have put into training it.

Yes, there is much to learn here but don't get distracted. Focus on learning one or two skills at a time until they have become strong, effortless, fluid and you have hardwired them into your brain so that they become your habitual way of moving. As time goes on you will further develop and refine these core skills so that you can generate more and more power with less and less effort.

The core skills are ones you will use all the time in almost all the kung fu skills you will learn. Never neglect them, practice them daily and make them a part of your life.

Adapt your exercises

Just like movement skills you can also adapt the exercises that you do. Some may otherwise be too hard or too easy or you don't have enough space to do them properly. Exercises can often be made easier or harder by changing the angle of the exercise or the amount of leverage required. In most of the exercises that follow I will give harder and easier examples but do feel free to experiment yourself, don't feel obliged to stick rigidly to my suggestions.

Another method of adaptation is to take a look around and see how you can adapt the things and environment around you to your training aims. I love taking everyday objects and using them to train my kung fu. This is the way kung fu has been trained forever - by using the environment and objects that came to hand.

The learning process

When you first learn a new exercise or combat movement your mind will struggle to coordinate your body effectively. You have roughly seven hundred muscles in the body although only around three hundred of those are involved in moving and stabilising your skeleton. Even so for each new movement you learn your brain needs to work out which muscles to fire and in what order, how far to contract each one and how powerful that contraction should be. That's an awful lot of calculations going on for even a simple movement. And bear in mind that most of our movements involve the whole body including weight being transferred from one leg to the other, a turning of the waist and some complicated movement of the arms and hands.

A lack of coordination is by far the biggest problem that newcomers to kung fu face.

Fortunately, your brain learns fast. After several repetitions, usually under a hundred, it will stumble on one that looks and feels about right. When that happens, it will store it in your memory like a mini program of that movement so that you never forget how to do it again. As they say, 'you never forget how to ride a bike'. You will also never forget how to perform a yang block or a back kick and so on.

That isn't the end of the story though, far from it. Even though you can 'do' a movement and remember it, the way that you do it is most likely inefficient. You will be using too much tension in certain muscles and underusing others. Only through endless repetitions can you gradually refine and hone each movement until it is as naturally powerful and effortless as can be.

You can 'learn' a new movement in one evening but it could take ten years to develop and perfect it.

You will also find that you 'learn' a new movement and are happy with it but then when you go to try it out on a partner all that learning goes out the window and you forget how to do it effectively. You end up focusing on your partner and trying to get them down in any way you can instead of focusing on yourself and your new-found movement skills. All your old bad habits come back to haunt you and you struggle unnecessarily to do the simplest things. This brings us on to the subject of partners.

Find a partner

You can only go so far with your training in this book unless you have regular access to at least one, preferably several people you can train with. This is the only way you can pressure test and fine tune your skills effectively. Ideally, you would go to a class run by a knowledgeable and enthusiastic instructor so that you could practice on a range of people but that isn't always possible or at least viable in many people's busy lifestyles.

Only partner training can give you the feedback you need so that you know you are on the right track. Every part of your kung fu training should be practised with a partner to test its effortless effectiveness. Obviously, there are elements where no partner is needed such as physical conditioning but for any combat skill a partner or two is going to push your training along so much faster. I will talk more about working with a partner later.

Chapter 9.
Stance Training

Stance training is the single most important element of good kung fu. Without good stances, your kung fu will be weak and worthless. Why is this?

Stance training is absolutely necessary to adapt your body to the workloads you make on it.

In kung fu a high emphasis is placed on developing a strong physical structure. That is the way in which the bones and muscles support each other so that any force applied to the body is absorbed throughout the body and not taken up by any one part of it. For example, any force taken up by the right arm is spread through the right arm and shoulder, down the back and uses the big muscles of the waist, hips and legs. Each of these muscles is used to create the force in the right arm and absorb the return force. Developing such a structure is a key part of general conditioning as it's something that you should learn to use all the time. Not just in kung fu practice but as part of your normal life as well. To learn to develop a good structure the first and most important factor is good stances.

Stances are the single most important element of training for all new students for at least the first year.

This is a view that has been shared by most major kung fu schools for centuries. In all those schools, stance training was focused on often to the exclusion of almost everything else for a long time. In many kung fu schools the new student would turn up and be forced to stand in the horse stance for as long as he could. Then he would be sent home. The next session it would be the same - standing in horse stance for as long as possible and then sent home. This would be continued for months to come. Gradually his legs would strengthen and his stance would lower. Only when he could stand in the stance for half an hour with a full cup of tea on his head, and another balanced on each arm and leg without spilling a drop was his stance considered acceptable. Only then would he begin martial training. By this time his legs were like steel and his body would be strong enough to receive or generate the forces necessary to withstand the training. Obviously, this kind of training wouldn't work in the West where people want instant results. Were schools to continue to try and train in this way they wouldn't have any students. So, stance training is mixed in with other skills to keep the classes more interesting for Westerners.

Stance training involves three main steps that will gradually give you the effortless power you seek. You don't need to focus on these steps separately, just standing in the stances will allow the changes to happen. However, it's worth having a look at these three steps to see what is going on.

Strengthen the legs

Most Westerners have weak legs due to spending most of their days sitting down. Strong legs are vital for good health as well as developing balanced power. It is the power of the legs that moves your body through all its movements. Even if you are just doing a small movement with one arm your legs should still be involved to support and power the arm movement. There are two kinds of leg training - training to support your body weight on increasingly bent legs and training to lift one leg in the air with balance and control. The stances give you a variety of ways to train both kinds of movement.

Relax the weight downwards

As you train your stances you will start to feel heavier and more stable. Throughout your stance training you should always aim to relax your whole bodyweight down through your legs and into the ground. As your legs become stronger you will feel a distinct dropping of the sacrum and the feeling that your legs are being pushed directly down into the ground. This shows that the weight of your upper body is now pushing directly through your legs into the ground.

Use the legs to carry the upper body

As your legs become stronger you will start to be able to carry more of the weight of your upper body in your legs. This sounds strange to most people who believe they are carrying their weight in their legs. Unfortunately, that isn't the case. Their weight is being carried from above by tension in the hips, chest, back and shoulders. This tension is there to carry the weight of the body as high as possible to take the strain out of weak legs. Stance training reverses this and strengthens the legs so that the upper body can release its tension and relax downwards. As your legs become strong and your upper body weight drops directly through them you can use them to directly power the movements of your arms and torso. It enables your upper body to remain loose and relaxed so that you aren't resisting your own movements with your shoulders, chest and back muscles. This lack of tension in your upper body means you can react quickly to changes in your opponent's movements and still generate enormous power as your arms are now directly connected to your very strong legs.

Stances don't just strengthen the legs. They also strengthen all the core muscles in the centre and up the back. Weak back muscles mean you have to lean forward to go deeper in the stances. As your back strengthens you can maintain a more upright position and the strong back will help to transfer and add to the power coming up from the legs.

One final note about stances - a stance describes the position of the legs, torso and head, in other words the entire body except for the arms. The arms are free to adopt a wide variety of positions from any stance.

Some of the descriptions for the stances, and other skills may differ from what you are used to. However, I will explain clearly why we do them this way and you should experiment for yourself to see which works best. I take nothing as read and have spent many years experimenting on hundreds of students and have complete faith in the efficacy of the various skills I present here.

Stability and the importance of pressure testing

I have had hundreds of students come to my school over the years. Many of them come from different martial backgrounds and many of them have trained stances before. Unfortunately, out of all those hundreds of students not one of them was able to stand in the horse stance - the most basic of stances without moving under pressure.

Many schools just get their students to stand in stances but never test them to see how stable they are.

Most schools don't even realise why they need to be stable which is odd as there is little point in stance training unless it is for stability. To understand the vital importance of this you need to understand some very simple physics.

Any force that builds up between two objects (ie two people in a fight) will always take the route of least resistance. In simple terms this means that if two people are pushing against each other it is not necessarily the strongest one who will win but the one who is the most stable. Quite often that is the strongest one as he may have more mass giving him more weight and his bigger muscles will give him a certain amount of stability.

Stance training gives you stability that weight training cannot. It specifically trains stability so that if someone pushes you they will not be able to move you. It also means that when you apply pressure to them such as with a strike or throw then the force will go into them and little or none of it will come back into you. Or to be more precise the force will come back into you but because of your stance training the force will naturally be directed through your body down into the ground. It won't move you backwards or cause any of your joints to give or collapse. This is where effortless power comes from.

It comes from stance training and nothing else can give it to you. Stance training also enables you to better withstand kicks and strikes and can make you almost invulnerable to throws.

Let's now take a look at the stances. In the system I teach we have eight stances. Some schools have more, some have less and it's likely that they may give them different names but often the stances will be largely the same. The five most useful and common stances are presented here. The other three will be in the next book.

The most important aspect of any stance is the bent knee. No power can be obtained from a straight leg.

Horse Stance

The most common and basic stance in all stance-based martial arts is the horse stance. Yet very few people can do it properly. Certainly, none of the hundreds of students I've taught, even those coming from martial arts backgrounds were able to stand and maintain an upright horse stance while someone pushes against them with all their force. It's perhaps the most important skill of all and can be learned in just five minutes yet not one of those students had ever been shown how. It would seem that this is knowledge that most martial arts schools lack yet it is so fundamental to making everything you do strong.

You can train in standing in stances for your whole life but you will never know if they are truly strong or not until you get somebody to push you while you stand in it. This is called pressure testing the stance and so few schools seem to pressure test their stances. Maybe it's because their stances don't stand up to being able to absorb force. Yet this is so important. With rock-solid stances, you can generate effortless power. Without them your body is disconnected and you struggle.

These are big statements but ones that have been borne out many times in sparring and partner practice in my classes. That's not to mention that they have proved their worth in centuries of real combat all across China. These principles are well known in the better kung fu schools but are rarely taught overtly. The traditional, 'Confucian' manner of teaching was such that principles were often left unexplained. If the student was worthy then he would be able to work them out for himself. This is the way I was taught and I guess I was worthy as I managed to work out the principles and physics of it myself. This knowledge I now pass on to you.

You should be testing your stances from the beginning. It's the only way to get the feedback you need to make the small adjustments necessary to make your stances totally strong. To test them effectively you need a partner. If you don't have a partner you can use a wall although a partner is better. I'll explain how to use a wall shortly.

To gain an immovable horse stance doesn't take years of practice as many may think or teachers may claim.

I have taught these principles to hundreds of students and every single one of them has managed to attain an immovable stance in less than five minutes. When I say immovable, I mean that I am able to push them with all my force and they don't move. It's just a question of following some simple principles. Let's start with the basics of the horse stance.

A horse stance is one where your weight is equally balanced between your feet which are shoulder length apart or wider. Your feet are facing forward and your knees are bent. Sit into the stance as if you were sitting on a horse, hence the name. Keep your head looking forward, not down, your back straight and your shoulders relaxed down. Now follow the principles below to make the stance immoveable.

Principle 1 - Align with gravity

This is the most important principle of all. You need to align your skeleton with all the forces that are acting on it.

In order to absorb or project force in the most efficient way your body must be balanced and holding on to the bare minimum of muscle tension. To achieve this your skeleton should be fully aligned with gravity so that your weight drops directly down through your feet and into the ground.

Any time you are leaning forward, even slightly or backward or sideways or your head is sticking forward

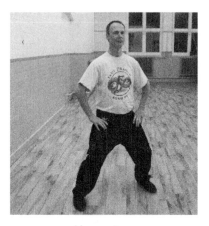

Horse stance

or your hips sticking backward there must be tension present in your muscles to stop you from falling over. This is tension that is lifting you up to stop you falling to the ground. It is tension that is not needed when you learn to stand properly upright. It's easy to be leaning forward, or more commonly backwards without even realising it so recruit a friend or stand side on to a mirror so that you can check your upper body is completely upright. After a while you won't need this as you will be able to feel when your body is properly aligned.

Tuck your hips under slightly so that your tailbone is pointing directly downwards. This will connect your legs to your upper body and makes a huge difference to your stability.

When your body is upright your muscles can relax around your skeleton and the weight of those relaxed muscles will root your body more firmly onto the ground

I cannot emphasise enough how important this is. As I tell my students, if you can't get this then you can't get anything. Forget about putting any real power in your techniques until you are able to align your body with gravity and feel when it isn't aligned.

Principle 2 - Relax downward

Now that you are upright and your skeleton is aligned with the downward pull of gravity relax downwards as much as you can. Let go of tension throughout your body and only allow as much as is necessary to stop you falling. With practice, you can let go of more and more tension. Indeed, one of the major benefits of stance training is the ability to release tensions that you don't need. This release of tension will enable you to handle the high levels of stress associated with combat. It will speed up your reflexes and movements and give you more control over every move you make. Areas to be aware of in particular are the hips and shoulders. These will take time to be able to relax properly but without relaxed hips your legs are disconnected from the torso. Without relaxed shoulders, your arms are on their own, disconnected from the rest of your body.

Principle 3 - Earth the force

In combat, there are at least two forces acting on your body: the constant pull of gravity plus the force that your opponent will be trying to apply to you. You have aligned yourself with gravity so now you need to align yourself to his or her changeable forces.

Imagine you are being pushed from the side. Now imagine a line from the point where this imaginary force is being applied that goes straight down to your opposite foot eg right shoulder to left foot and into the earth. Feel the force following through that imaginary line downwards but don't allow that line to collapse. You will probably feel a slight shift in your muscles as your body prepares for force to be applied from that side. You are developing a 'ground path' – a direct line of force from the ground to any part of your body.

Pressure test the stance

Now it's time to try it for real. Find a partner and ask them to push into your shoulder from the side. Get them to start with just a little pressure while you get used to directing it down into the earth. Do not push back into them or collapse at all. Stay upright, stay balanced and stay relaxed. To start with they will be able to feel your body give as they push. When you can direct the force downwards they should be able to push into you with all their force and you can stay relaxed yet not be moved at all. To them it will feel as if they were pushing directly into the earth. This is key knowledge that is rarely explained in books or videos.

It can also help to try pressure testing mistakes. For example, try tensing your muscles or sticking your bum out slightly. Either of these will make you very easy to push over. They will show you how important it is to relax and get the small details right.

If you can't find a partner try it with a wall. Pressure testing against walls or other immovable objects is always good practice. Stand a foot or so away from a wall sideways onto it so that you can reach out to the side with your right palm and push it. If you have followed the principles correctly you should be able to push the wall hard and not move at all. Yet if you are even slightly out of alignment, even a gentle push will be enough to move you. Experiment with different positions to see which is the most rooted and also to see how easy it is to move you even when you are only slightly misaligned.

Note that the horse stance is very stable if pushed from the side. But if someone pushes you from the front or back it is far less stable, at least without lots of practice and the right principles to follow. It can be developed to be stable but that is more advanced and will be covered in a future book. As the stance is inherently less stable from a forward or backward force it is clearly not a good idea to punch directly forward from a horse stance. However, this is routinely seen in martial arts films and is done in countless classes around the world.

Why punch from an unstable stance? It's no good asking me as I don't do it but if you go to a class that does you should ask your own teacher. The horse stance is virtually useless for any move that involves forward or backward power. It is good for side to side power or taking someone directly down, for throws or balanced upward force etc. It is also unparalleled for training the legs, just don't try to punch forward with it. The only exception for this is if you twist your body to one side to strike with the other fist - i.e. twisting to the left to strike with the right fist. This can generate a lot of power but your body is still in the wrong position for the return force which will knock you backwards.

Horse stance pointers

- Feet at least shoulder width apart.
- Knees bent and sit into the stance.
- Weight equally balanced between feet.
- Upper body upright and relaxed down.
- Hips tucked slightly under.

- Align your body with gravity and the forces that your opponent is applying.

The principles of being upright, aligned with gravity and relaxed down apply equally to all the stances. In fact, they should also be applied to everything you do throughout your whole life.

Dragon Stance

The dragon stance is the second major power stance in most kung fu styles. Where the horse stance gives maximum stability when force is applied from the side the dragon stance gives stability when force is applied from the front. In some styles, it may be called the front stance or the bow and arrow stance.

To see in which direction you or your opponent are strongest simply draw an imaginary line from one foot to the other. That is the line of power and on that axis or near it they will be stable. However, if you apply force at an angle perpendicular to it they will be weak and vulnerable to attack. This is why it's not a good idea to punch forward from a horse stance (which you see in almost all martial arts films). To show how unstable it can be stand in a horse stance in front of a wall and push into the wall and see just how easily you'll be pushed backwards. The best stance for applying power to the front of your body is the one we call the dragon stance.

The dragon stance is important because when you are applying a forceful forward movement such as a power strike it is the stance you will end up in. It ensures your body is completely stable at the critical point of impact so all the impact force will go into your opponent and you won't be unbalanced or moved by it.

How to do it

To stand in the dragon stance step one foot in front of the other but slightly out to one side so that you have some stability left to right.

Bend your front knee so that your lower leg is vertical and straighten, or nearly straighten your back leg. Your back foot should be turned out no more than 45 degrees otherwise you run the risk of twisting your ankle should you suddenly receive force from the front. Make sure your back heel is on the floor and stays on the floor. All too often when punching the weight goes too far forward and the back heel comes up which destroys your stability. When you are punching forward or applying any force to the front relax your weight down through your back foot to counter the forward force of the hand. But remember not to lean backwards or forwards while doing this.

Another point is not to make the stance too long. In karate, they use long stances as a longer stance lowers your body weight and makes you more stable. However, you pay for that with a lack of mobility - in other words it's hard to get out of a long stance quickly. Everything in combat is a trade-off between mobility and stability. The more mobile you are in any position the less stable you are and vice versa. The Chinese of antiquity solved that dilemma by learning how to direct force into the ground so they could maintain fairly high stances which were mobile and yet still be stable. If your stance is too long to move out of quickly it is too long. Mobility is more important than stability for 90% of the time in combat. The stance should only be slightly longer than your normal walking step.

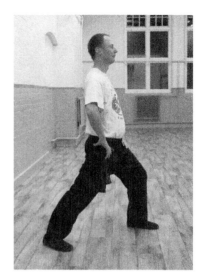

Dragon stance

Make sure your hips are square to the direction you're facing. Extend your arms forward, if they are the same length then your hips are square. With hips square to the attacker you can use either arm to attack or defend. If the hips aren't square you can only use your leading arm.

The stability in the legs needs to be transferred to the arms so, with your arms extended out in front of you, mentally push your arms slightly forward while at the same time, relaxing/pushing your back leg into the ground. Also tuck your hips under to firmly connect your upper body to your lower body.

When you can step forward into this position comfortably and accurately it's time to pressure test it. In this position, you should easily be able to withstand the force of someone pushing into your hands with all their weight and strength without collapsing backwards.

The dragon stance pointers

- Front leg bent, back leg straight.

- Hips square to the front.

- A gap between the legs, not one directly in front of the other.

- Hips tucked slightly under.

- Back foot facing forward or nearly forward. Certainly, no more than 45 degrees out to the side and make sure your heel stays on the floor.

- Don't make the stance too long.

- Upper body upright and relaxing downwards

Tiger Stance

The tiger stance is another great stance to develop leg strength. Most of the weight is on the back leg so it enables you to move forward with power. It is also great practice to move from a tiger stance forward into a dragon stance and back to tiger. The back foot will need repositioning as I shall explain.

To learn to stand in the tiger stance start off in the horse stance. Move some of your weight onto your right leg then turn your left foot and leg outward ninety degrees. Keep your knees apart and feet facing the same direction as your thighs. Turn your upper body in the direction of your left foot. As with the dragon stance above with your arms extended out in front of you, mentally push your arms slightly forward while at the same time, relaxing/pushing your back leg into the ground. This mental connection between your arms and legs is essential in developing whole-body power.

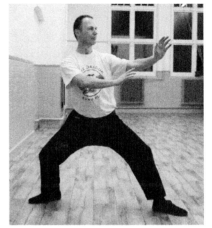

Tiger stance

The chambered fist

Often you will see someone in a tiger stance in films, videos or images and the leading arm is extended as it should be but their back fist is held at the hip. Why is this? In combat, the correct place for both of your hands is between yourself and your opponent, or opponents as in the picture above.

Having one hand held at your hip is all but useless to you, you might as well tie it behind your back. However, a great number of martial arts schools teach this as standard. If you ask them why they do it the reason you will hear is that the punch is 'chambered' at the hip to give the punch more power. Yes, you may get slightly more power by driving it forward and pulling the other fist back by using torque through the upper body. This does work but there are better ways to do so that don't put one of your arms in an unusable position. The downside of the 'chambered fist' is that your fist is placed in a position where it can't defend you. Not only that but any attacker can plainly see that it is chambered at the hip and so is likely to strike forward. He will be expecting your punch and by the time you have driven it forward from your hip into its target he will have seen the move and blocked or avoided it.

If you attack in a predictable way you will get a predictable outcome'.

There are times when you will punch from the hip but the attacking fist should never be held at the hip first. If you have your arms by your side and wish to make a sudden forward punch your hand would come up to the hip first by bending at the elbow then your fist would be driven forward in a powerful forward strike. This would be done in exactly the same way it used to be done in Western films where two cowboys would stand facing each other and the fastest draw would shoot the other one. The hand shoots up to the hip to grab the gun then, without stopping, shoots forward to fire or, in this case, punch. The hip is part of the route the fist would take to get to its target, but shouldn't be the starting point where it is obvious to your opponent what your intentions are.

There is one good reason to hold the fist at the hip but it is not for striking. The only good reason to hold a closed hand at the hip is when it is holding onto your opponent's arm or wrist and has pulled them back into a position where you can apply a strike, lock or throw. This is the real reason why you see the hand at the hip in so many forms but it has been widely misinterpreted as being held ready to strike. This is just one of many ways in which so many forms have lost much of their original meaning and been misinterpreted to such an extent that they are barely usable any more.

Tiger stance pointers

- Front foot facing forward.
- Rear foot facing 90 degrees or slightly more out to the side.
- Both knees bent, back leg more than front leg.
- Sixty percent or more weight on the back leg.
- Knees apart and feet flat on the floor.
- Hips tucked slightly under.
- Upper body upright and relaxing downward.

Cat Stance

When you first stand in the cat stance it seems to be an inherently unstable position to stand in. This is because all your weight is resting on one leg with the other leg just resting under its own weight on the ground. Yet in most of the kung fu styles I teach this is the most important stance of all and the one my more advanced students spend the most time in. So, what makes this stance so special?

Firstly, and most importantly is the question of mobility. In the cat stance, all the body-weight is on the back leg. This means the front foot is free to move in any direction it pleases. When your body is driven forward from the bent back leg it has to move in the direction of the front foot. So, keeping your weight off the front foot means you can change direction quickly. If you were double-weighted, i.e. your weight was equally balanced between your feet, you would have to get your weight off one of your feet before you could move it. This wastes time and time is measured by milliseconds in combat. In the cat stance, your unweighted front foot contains a lot of potential. It can move further forward or sideways or backward or raise into a kick instantaneously.

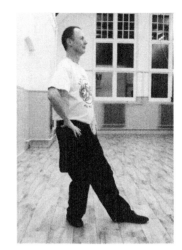

From a defensive point of view, the cat stance lets you turn away from an incoming attack quickly. If somebody goes for a straight-line punch or grab you just put your weight on one leg and turn the hips in the direction of the unweighted foot. Now you are in the cat stance and your entire body is out of the line of attack.

Finally, the cat stance is the best stance if someone is pulling you from the front although the tiger stance is also good for this. If you want to pull someone back and down just grab them then take a small step back and drop your weight down onto your back leg.

Cat stance

In many kung fu styles the cat stance is the most important stance of all.

Cat stance pointers

- All your weight should be on your back leg. You should be able to lift your front foot and not fall forward.

- Your back foot can be facing forward or up to 90 degrees out to the side. A position of around 45 degrees to the front foot is usually best for balance and mobility.

- As always, your hips should be tucked under slightly and your upper body kept upright and relaxing downwards.

- Raise the chest and sink the back.

This stance will feel unstable and unbalanced to start with. But with practice you will be able to resist someone pushing you from the front with force without falling backwards and while maintaining all the attributes of the stance.

Crane Stance

The crane stance is another widely known stance and simple to do. You just lift one leg up in the air and keep it there. It sounds simple but, of course it isn't. Certain parts of your body need to be stable while others need to be able to move slightly to enable you to adjust your balance to the pull of gravity. The crane stance is mostly for developing your legs for kicking.

Crane stance attributes

- Stand on one leg with the other knee raised as high as possible
- Standing leg bent at the knee
- Raised foot pointing downwards, not flexed

There are three other stances we use in this system - the scissor stance, kneeling stance and snake stance but I will talk more about those in the next book.

Remember to practice all your stances regularly.

Each stance will develop your legs in a different way. Over time you will go through the process of 'burning in' your stances. This process takes a few months and to start with your legs will ache, a lot. Then they will start to shake, then they start to burn. Eventually the sensation goes away and you can stand comfortably for a long time in the stance.

Also, over time you should try to lower the height of your stances. You bend your knees more and focus on dropping your hips i.e. releasing tension in your lower back. As your legs get stronger you will take more of the weight from your upper body directly in the legs so you will be less tense in the chest, back, neck and shoulders. You will become increasingly immoveable in your stances and every technique you do will have added power that is coming up from your legs. You will be able to drop down into low stances and spring up again into high ones instantly. This will make you less predictable and can confuse attackers. The monkey style specialises in this type of movement.

So, whatever practice time you have available spend half of it standing in these stances. Of that stance time spend half of it standing in the horse stance with the other half divided among the other stances. Do that until you can stand easily in a fairly deep horse stance for *at least* fifteen minutes. Even then don't abandon your stance training or you will get gradually weaker. Later on in this book, you will find exercises to do with your arms while you are standing in your stances.

Teaching of these stances and many other skills are available at the online training section of our school website -
www.jadedragonschool.com

Chapter 10.

Bodyweight Exercises

Everybody comes to kung fu with a different level of fitness. Some people are regular gym goers or have studied other sports or martial arts. Some people start kung fu having lived a sedentary life until then.

Kung fu requires a certain base level of strength in the main muscle groups and that strength is then multiplied many times by learning to connect the body together efficiently. Even without a base level of strength learning to use your body in a connected way will make you stronger than most people could believe but adding basic strengthening exercises will naturally add to that power.

Strangely, the main reason for adding strengthening exercises isn't necessarily to make you stronger. It is to give you a more balanced musculature. Most humans have particularly weak legs and a weak back. Stance training will strengthen the legs and back but it is a static exercise and to balance the stances require exercises that move the body through a range of motion.

It is better to use your own bodyweight as resistance rather than weights, at least until your body is balanced.

Adding weights too soon can put intolerable strain on a skeletal system. Particularly if it is being constantly pulled out of alignment by tension.

There is a school of thought prevalent among those who practice t'ai chi chuan and some other 'internal' martial arts that you shouldn't do any external strength training. They say that doing so causes excess tension in the muscles and they are aiming for complete relaxation. They also say that strength training interferes with energy flow. This, I believe to be a common misconception and a misunderstanding of old teachings.

Firstly, and perhaps most importantly, the people who lived in feudal China when these practices were developed did not live the sedentary lives that modern Westerners do. They already had a much stronger and more flexible physique from the manual work they had to do each day. I believe the teachings told them that their own level of strength was enough and they should focus their attention on making the body more balanced, relaxed and connected rather than trying to strengthen individual muscles further. Secondly there was a misunderstanding about the Chinese word Sung. It is commonly translated to mean relaxed but that isn't really a good description of it.

In the West when we think of being relaxed we think of having no tension at all. The word Sung doesn't mean limp and lifeless but it means holding no excess tension, being in a state that is neither tense nor completely limp. If you can imagine cutting a rubber band so that it is one piece of rubber and holding it at one end. The part of the band that is hanging down will curl up in different ways due to the internal tensions in the rubber. That is lifeless and useless. Now hold the other end and straighten the band but without stretching it. Now the band is what the Chinese call Sung. It is capable of transmitting force or chi energy from one end to the other yet without tensing up unduly.

So, the word Sung means to be relaxed yet alert and ready to move instantly. It doesn't mean a state of complete relaxation which loses connection between the body parts.

A sedentary lifestyle mirrors that of a cut rubber band. Some parts of the body are too weak and others are too tight. The body is pulled this way and that and there is little coordinating organisation of the body parts. Some kinds of physical exercise such as bodyweight training make the body work against itself and improve coordination of agonistic and antagonistic muscles and body parts. Agonists being parts of the body that work together such as quads and hip flexors. Antagonists work against each other such as biceps and triceps.

Bodyweight training is superior to weight training as weights, particularly weight machines, force the body to move in unnatural ways. This can, and often does, cause injury in certain joints, particularly in the shoulders and knees which are susceptible to these kinds of injuries. From personal experience, I would say that bodyweight training coupled with static power exercises is the way forward for the newcomer to kung fu. Over time you will not just become stronger but you will gain more control over your muscles and all the other parts of your body. Your body and mind will then work together to produce extraordinary results.

In this chapter is a selection of bodyweight exercises designed to strengthen your body in a natural way. When performing the exercises below keep in mind the following:

- When learning a new exercise start off slowly. Keep well within your limits and let your body learn the new exercise and adapt to it before trying to increase it. Otherwise you will find yourself in pain and not making the progress you want.

- It is not necessarily the amount of reps and sets you can do that count. It is the overall length of time you spend with your muscles under strain. Being able to do 30 fast press-ups that you can do in 20 seconds is not going to be as beneficial as doing 10 slow press-ups that take 4 seconds each to complete. The slower pace means your muscles are under strain for longer and you are having to control them every inch of the way rather than using gravity on the way down and momentum on the way up.

- Form is extremely important and by form I mean posture and alignment. If your posture isn't good then the forces of the movement will take unpredictable paths through your body and you could end up injuring weaker muscles that had to take the force unexpectedly. Once you have gained some power in these exercises you can also make them harder by trying them on a less predictable surface such as trying press ups on a gym ball.

- Work within your limits but aim to increase the number of reps and sets gradually. A rep is a repetition for example one full press-up. A set is a group of reps such as one set of ten press-ups then a rest followed by another set of ten. If you struggle to do one full rep successfully then adapt the movement to make it easier. If you can do several sets in good form of an exercise with ease then adapt it to make it harder. I will give suggestions for adaptations as we go along.

Squats

The average person associates strength with power in the upper body - bulging shoulders, pecs and biceps. But real power in kung fu comes from having strong legs and being able to transfer the power of the legs up into the arms and hands. In kung fu all movements of the upper body rely on forces transmitted through the legs. The stance training I covered earlier teaches you how to transfer the force of the upper body down into the legs and back up. Just standing in the positions and relaxing into the ground does that automatically.

Strong legs make everything else you do easier. The sedentary lifestyles that we are almost forced to lead causes us to spend at around 90% of our day sitting or lying down. This prevents us from building and maintaining leg muscle and is wholly unnatural for us as a species. We evolved to walk for long periods, to run, to climb and to squat. Before the invention of chairs people used to sit on the ground or squat as a way of resting their legs. Legs were used all day every day. In kung fu the power of all of your movements starts from the legs.

Many adults in the East retain the ability to squat easily. It is a natural resting position for them

Weak legs directly cause tension in the upper body in an attempt to take some of the weight off the legs. Weak leg muscles are not able to adequately support the knee and hip joints so these joints weaken and become painful as we age. They also become far more prone to injury as the muscles aren't strong enough to maintain the integrity of the joint in the case of a sudden impact.

There is one exercise that trains all the muscles in the legs beyond all others. It is probably the oldest and simplest leg exercise in the world - we call it the squat. Squats can be done anytime, anywhere with no need for special equipment.

The squat is an exercise that lowers the torso by bending the joints at the hips, knees and ankles. A proper squat works every single muscle, large and small in the hips and legs. It also works the lower back and abdominal muscles as well which are used to keep the upper body stable during the movement.

How to do it

To perform the basic squat stand with your feet shoulder width apart or slightly wider. Your feet can be pointing slightly outwards but no more than the angle of your upper legs. Now bend slowly at the hips and knees down to the natural limit of your movement, pause for a few seconds and then slowly raise up again. This pause at the lowest point of the movement enables you to relax into that position and gradually your hips and ankle joints will open up and allow you to sit deeper into the stance.

Do as many reps as you are able to, rest and then do some more. Aim to do at least two sets of squats every day if you want strong legs. If you find full squats hard at first then hold onto the back of a chair or similar support to help you down and up.

Points to remember:

- Keep your back straight throughout the movement

- Don't push your knees forward but keep the knees at the same point in space and squat down behind them

- Don't lift your heels off the floor. This will interfere with your stability and put too much tension through the knees. If your calves and achilles tendon are too tight then focus on stretching them first. Gradually they will open up and you can go lower

- Make the movement as full as possible - go down as far as is possible with a straight back and feet flat on the floor, then all the way back up again. Do this slowly and under full control.

- Experiment with different arm positions. Straight out in front of you is probably the best as it gives some counter weight to the exercise. I also enjoy squatting with fingers held lightly behind the head and elbows drawn backward as this lifts the chest and strengthens the upper back.

Squatting involves the use of all the biggest muscles in your body. Therefore, it is a hard exercise to do. If you feel that unsupported squatting is too much for you to start with then hold on to something as you raise and lower your body. This will give extra support and enable you to help your legs by slightly pushing down with your arms as you raise back up to the standing position. However, don't rely on this and progress to unsupported squatting as soon as you can.

Squat progressions

Squats are easily the best leg strengtheners there are so there will come a time when you are finding them too easy to do and have to do a lot of repetitions to get the benefit. Most people at this point will be tempted to try to add extra weight by holding dumbbells or squatting with a weighted rucksack or such like. There is no need to hold any additional weights as you squat as these can put intolerable strain on the spine.

To make the movement harder use one of the progressions below.

Circular squats

With your feet in the same position as the standard squat above bring your weight more over your left leg and slowly squat down. Then transfer your weight to the right leg and slowly come up. Then squat down on the right leg and up on the left. Repeat as necessary.

Close squats

This is performed in the same way as the standard squat but the feet are closer together. Over time you can bring the feet together and still perform full squats. This increases the load on the quadriceps and strengthens the knees, shins and gluteals.

Uneven squats

Stand as in the basic squat but with one foot resting firmly on a basketball or similar. The leg that is on the ground is now forced to do most of the work so do several reps on this leg then swap the ball to the other leg. This is the progression towards the full one legged squat. Over time, stretch the supported leg out in front of you and then try it without support gradually going lower until you can achieve a full one legged squat.

Squat every day and your legs, hips, back and abdomen will soon become strong and your whole posture will change. It will do wonders for your kung fu skills.

Push Ups

The push-up or press-up really is the ultimate upper body exercise. It powerfully coordinates the arms to work with the midsection and trains the chest, shoulders, triceps and abs in a way that is functional and doesn't put excess strain though the joints.

There are many variations of the push-up and they each work the muscles slightly differently but they all provide great strength and muscle building benefits. Apart from the chest, shoulders and arms that all get a good workout through the correct range of movement, the push-up also trains many other muscles isometrically. These are the muscles that are holding the body in place in order to perform the movement. These other muscles include the lats, the spinal muscles, the deeper chest muscles, the abdomen, the waist and the quads.

How to do it

The press-up is such an easy exercise to understand and perform. Just lie prone on the floor and push yourself up with your hands. Then lower yourself until you are just above the floor and push up again and again.

Points to remember:

- Stick to regular push ups until you are used to the movement and can do at least 2 sets of 15 with ease.

- Work at keeping your whole body aligned, you may need a mirror to check this. Sagging in the middle or raising the hips just shows that your core muscles aren't yet strong enough to hold you in position.

- Keep your feet together. This makes the exercise harder as you are now using extra muscles to stabilise your body as you raise and lower. These muscles are essential for your kung fu.

- Don't forget to breathe. Try not to hold your breath at all during the movements but keep your breathing slow and even.

- Perform each push up slowly. Take at least one second to go down and another to come up again. Try pausing at the bottom of each rep and tensing the triceps at the top. This will build strength much faster as you are controlling your weight all the way down and up and not relying on momentum.

When you are comfortable with your push ups and are looking for more variety then try the following.

- Change your hand position. Move your hands further apart or closer together. Or keep them higher or lower than shoulder height on the floor. Each of these variations will use different muscle fibres to take up the work.

- Turn your hands slightly out on the ground so your thumbs are pointing forward and keep your elbows in close to your side during the press-ups.

- Take more of the weight on one arm or the other. You could try lowering down on mostly one arm, transferring the weight to the other arm and pushing up on it then change direction. This will help you towards the possibility of one armed pushups.

- Change the hand shape. Try doing pushups on the backs of your hands, your knuckles (holdng a fist) or your fingertips. These will strengthen that part of your hand for striking. A word of caution though - don't do knuckle push ups on a hard surface as it will eventually wreck your knuckles. They are fine on a carpet or on grass but not on a hard floor.

Start your push up training today. It will strengthen any movement that involves pushing or punching forward. It will also train that important power chain from feet to hands.

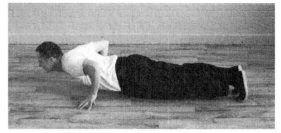

Fingertip pushups

Pull Ups

We are apes. We may be standing on just two legs and be more follically challenged than other apes but we are still apes. This means that we have spent millions of years evolving to be good at climbing trees. Over the last six million years or so, which is just a brief period in evolutionary terms, the need for us to pull ourselves up onto tree branches has greatly diminished. This lack of exercise for our back is yet another reason why we are posturally unbalanced with weak backs and sore shoulders.

The pullup, like the push-up is a natural exercise that doesn't force the joints into any unnatural positions. It develops power in the back muscles and also in the shoulders, abdomen and biceps. It also greatly increases your grip strength which is important in many martial arts.

Remember that pull-ups is an exercise that we have evolved to do.
Few exercises should be more natural to us.

All training should be balanced. If you do a lot of push training e.g. pushups or bench presses then you need to balance this out with pull training and the most effective and natural of these is the pullup. Otherwise the muscles at the front of your shoulder will become too strong and move the shoulder joint out of alignment. This will lead to pain and decreased mobility as you age. Apart from anything else strong back muscles enable you to create awesome down force which is something all martial artists should aspire to. The deep back muscles take over many arm movements from the shoulder muscles enabling you to release tension in the arms. This means that they can move with more speed and fluid ease yet without sacrificing any power.

How to do it

Clearly before you start you will need a pullup bar. If you don't have one you can buy a pullup bar which hooks over a door frame. This is what I use. The only problem with these is that it is impossible to let your legs hang all the way down as the floor is in the way. The other alternative is one that screws into the wall and is just higher than you can reach up with fingers outstretched.

The full body weight pullup is a challenging exercise which you are unlikely to be able to do unless you have done some preparatory training first. The best way to start is to use your legs to aid the upward movement. In other words take a comfortable grip on your bar with hands shoulder width or more apart. Then place your feet on a stable base such as a stool or table and use your feet to aid the upward pull of your arms.

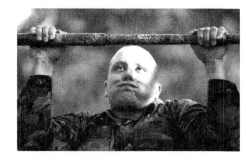

Obviously, you want to use your legs as little as possible, doing most of the work with your arms. Don't think of this as cheating, it is the first stage of the process of increasing your back, bicep, and grip strength. Remember, this is an exercise that you were designed to do so your back will quickly build power (and width).

Be patient with yourself and through consistent training you should soon find yourself able to achieve your first full bodyweight pullup. Mark this day on your exercise log and now you can set about increasing the reps you are able to do.

Points to remember

- As with all strength exercises your aim should be to perform each movement slowly so as to use muscle power rather than momentum.

- Use your legs as little as possible and focus your attention on your back and arms.

- Once you are able to perform full pullups resist the temptation to make up thrusting movements with your knees to help yourself get up to manage a final rep or two. This is defeating the purpose of strengthening your upper body. Use muscle power in the arms and back only.

- At the bottom of the movement keep your back tight. Don't allow your shoulders to relax all the way as this will put strain on the ligaments and can damage the shoulders. Maintain a slight downward force in the shoulder blades and a slight bend in the elbows.

Buy a pullup bar and start your pullup training today.

Leg Raises

Abdominal exercises remain one of the most popular types of exercise as everyone wants a flat, even a ripped stomach. Abdominal exercises are all over the internet and on the front of most fitness magazines. This is all well and good to a point but there are two problems with most abdominal exercises. Firstly, it isn't possible to lose fat from a particular area just by exercising the muscles in this area. This has been known for years but still doesn't stop exercise magazines from promoting the latest ab crunch workout on their front covers in the expectation that people with a lot of belly fat will believe it and buy them.

If you are carrying excess fat around your middle your abs will only start to show when your fat levels decrease below a certain point. The only real way to get them there is simple - it's to eat less carbs, particularly processed and sugary foods. I have never been in any way overweight but I once gave up sugar completely for six weeks and went from a 34" waist to a 31" waist without making any other changes or giving anything else up. I ate an awful lot of nuts during that time.

In fact, having a ripped stomach is not a priority in kung fu but having strong core strength most certainly is. This leads us to the second problem with most abdominal exercises. The most commonly promoted exercise for the abdomen - the crunch or sit-up is *not* the best exercise for developing a strong abdominal core.

If you want a truly powerful midsection, and as a kung fu artist you really do, then the leg raise is the way to go. The leg raise is far more effective than any ab crunch you have done before. It trains not just the central abdomen but all the muscles of the waist: the obliques, the transverse, psoas, intercostals and serratus. These muscles provide a solid midsection that can generate great force that is transferred directly to the arms and legs for real power delivery.

Most of the movements in kung fu rely on force being transmitted through powerful legs and a powerful midsection out to the arms. Any force coming from the front would bend the body backwards without powerful abdominal muscles. Many kung fu skills rely on turning the waist for power. The more powerful those oblique muscles are along with the rest of the midsection the more powerful each of those skills will be.

The leg raise doesn't just train killer abs but also powerful leg raising force for jumping or kicking. It trains all the muscles needed to lift the knee and push the leg outwards into a kick. It isn't just the leg muscles involved but the core as well and the leg raise is the exercise to train the whole area. It is a far superior exercise to the crunch which only trains part of the chain of muscles and then fairly weakly. The crunch was invented by steroid taking bodybuilders to gently tone the stomach area without adding thickness to their 'roid gut'. This is an enlarged gut that's a side-effect from taking steroids. The last thing they wanted were effective abdominal exercises that would strengthen and thicken the abdominal area further so they invented this gentle toning exercise, the crunch.

If you aren't taking performance enhancing drugs, and I hope you aren't, then crunches are not the best ones for your core training. Not only that but your abs were not designed to crunch, twist, and bend as they do in all crunching exercises. In fact, it's the complete opposite! The real role of your abdominal muscles is to prevent your mid-section from crunching, twisting, and bending. That's right, your abs are a stabilising force designed to resist spinal movement in order to protect your spine. They're also involved in shortening in order to raise the knees hence the point of this exercise.

How to do it

There are two kinds of leg raises - the easier supine leg raise and the more challenging hanging leg raise.

The supine leg raise

1. Start in the supine position (lying on your back)

2. Lie flat on the floor (on a mat) place your arms out to the side on the floor with your palms facing down.

3. Make sure that your head, legs and lower back are all in contact with the floor.

4. Engage your stomach muscles.

5. Bend your knees and slowly lift your legs to a 90-degree angle or more if you can,

6. Pause for a second then slowly lower the legs back down.

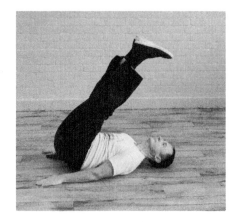

When you can comfortably do 10 or more of these then gradually straighten the legs until you can easily do 10 or more with your legs completely straight. Do not allow your lower back to lift off the floor. It is your abdominal muscles that are being used to push it down there.

The hanging leg raise

When you can comfortably do 2-3 sets of straight legged raises then you are ready for the more difficult hanging leg raise. For this you will need a hanging bar. You can buy bars that fit over door frames or go all out and get one that is screwed into the wall.

With hanging leg raises your abs and hip flexors are lifting the full weight of your legs up in the air. So again start with bent knees and gradually progress until you can do full straight legged hanging leg raises. By that time you will have abs of steel. If you're female don't worry, you won't look like that but will still have a very toned and powerful core midsection.

Make leg raises a regular part of your weekly schedule and all your other exercises and movements will be stronger because of it.

The Flying Crane

The flying crane exercise strengthens all the muscles of the back and aids with balance at the same time. It is a traditional exercise in some kung fu styles.

Back strength is as crucial a component of kung fu as it is of life. Most people have weak backs as we don't use them for most of the day as we are resting them on the back of chairs. Even while standing the back muscles are only weakly engaged and cannot compete with the gradual shortening of the front of the body. As we age we tend to lean forward because of our weak back muscles. Back pain is one of the most common reasons people go to see their doctor but if their backs were strong enough to meet the demands of everyday life they wouldn't need the painkillers and eventual surgery that so many millions have to endure.

Every time you extend an arm or leg out in front of you there needs to be compensatory tension in the back muscles. The stronger your back is the more power you can generate in the front of your body, it is that simple. Many people struggle with lifting weights or pushing something heavy but their limitation isn't necessarily in the chest, arms or abdomen but in their weak back muscles. In India, they say that a man's age is measured by the age of his spine. Learn to strengthen your back today and you will feel the benefits almost instantly.

The flying crane is a seemingly simple exercise yet it has many and profound benefits. It strengthens your hamstrings, glutes (buttock muscles), lower and upper back, back of shoulder and back of neck muscles. The body rotates around its central axis in the lower abdomen - an area known in China as the dantian. This teaches you to properly connect the power of the legs and the back muscles with fluid strength. You can add a forward component to further strengthen the abdomen and chest at the same time.

How to do it.

1. Stand with your feet close together and your arms by your sides.

2. Bring your weight onto your right foot and slowly raise your left leg into the air behind you. Keep the leg straight at the knee.

3. At the same time lean forward to counter the weight of the raised leg behind you and extend your arms out to shoulder height. This is the final position.

4. Hold for a second or two then return slowly back to the start by lowering the leg, raising the body back to the vertical and lowering your arms. Then repeat a few more times also repeating the same number of reps on the other leg.

If you wish you can perform the move then, without allowing your raised foot to touch the floor, bring it back up into a crane stance and bring your arms in front of you and press your palms together. Then move back into flying crane position. This will strengthen the whole core and add immeasurably to your balance and poise at the same time.

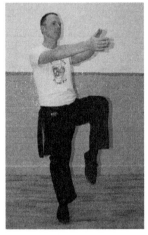

Raise leg into crane stance and extend arms in front

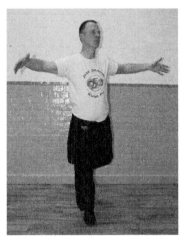

Slowly bring leg back behind you and extend arms out and back

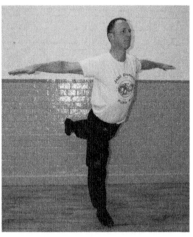

Extend arms and leg fully back and lift chest and head

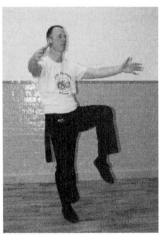

Slowly bring leg and arms back to front

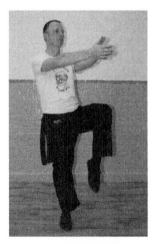

Return to beginning position and repeat

Points to remember

- Keep your back leg straight at the knee when you raise it behind you.

- Lift your chest as you lean forward and try to arch your back backwards.

- Keeping your supporting knee bent will aid with balance and stability.

Having a strong back is vital to kung fu and to life. The flying crane will get you started on that journey. Another even more fabulous exercise for the back is the bridge. The flying crane will start to work the key muscles you need to perform a true back bridge so I'll cover that further in my next book.

Chapter 11.
Flexibility and Mobility

Flexibility is an important aspect of gaining a healthy body and of particular importance to anyone wishing to learn kung fu. In the West, we consider cardiovascular exercise to be the cornerstone of any exercise system but in the East flexibility is given that honour. I also believe that flexibility is more important than cardio for maintaining a fit and healthy body.

For many decades now we, in the West have been consistently told that the most important element of fitness, the one thing we all need to focus our energies on, is cardiovascular training – in other words, stamina. We are told this is good for the heart – hence the word cardio, we are told this will help us lose weight by burning off our fat and so on.

In the East, they believe that flexibility is much more important than stamina when it comes to human health.

Why flexibility is king

The biggest triggers for ill health in the developed world are stress, obesity and diabetes. You can link obesity and diabetes together as by and large they have the same cause – an excessive intake of empty calories from sugar and other highly processed foods. So how does flexibility training measure up to cardiovascular training in combating the ills of the modern world?

Cardiovascular training works by strengthening the heart muscle and pushing blood around the system. The warmed-up muscles feel more relaxed and you burn off calories during and after the workout.

Flexibility exercises work by stretching your muscles and other soft tissue which have become shortened and hardened from lack of movement. These flexible soft tissues improve your posture and release tension in your muscles so that blood can flow through them more easily.

This is an important point. If you find that water isn't flowing freely through your pipes at home is it best to upgrade the pumping mechanism or to locate and clear out any blockages?

Stretching releases tension in the muscles that is preventing and blocking efficient blood flow. This, in turn, reduces blood pressure and takes a lot of strain off the heart. Flexibility returns your body back to a state of balance. The benefits of flexibility are way more than simply increasing range of movement and blood flow.

Most people are carrying huge burdens of tension in the majority of muscles in their body. This pulls them in different directions all the time, bending their posture out of shape and requiring large amounts of energy to maintain. A regular stretching regime releases that tension allowing the body to return to a posture that can be aligned with gravity and so move with maximum efficiency. Moreover, it requires a lot less energy and effort to maintain or move a posture that has minimal tension. In short, you gain far more control over your body and will have more energy available for everyday life.

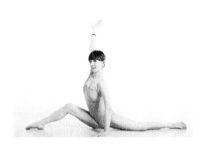

The more flexible you are, the more you are able to relax. The more you are able to relax, then the easier flexibility is to attain. It is a virtuous circle.

From a sport or martial arts point of view flexibility will help prevent you from injury and will speed up recovery from muscle soreness after a hard training session. It also gives you the range of movement necessary to perform your sport or martial art effectively without struggling against your own limitations.

Finally, it acts as an accurate barometer of your stress levels. When you know how far you can go in any particular stretch you can easily determine how stressed you are by trying that stretch to see how far you can get. Some days it will be fairly easy but when you're stressed or tired your range of movement could be halved.

Tiredness itself usually comes from the build-up of tension in your body. This tension wears you out as you're constantly fighting against it.

Hard and soft tension

Anybody who is used to stretching exercises will be familiar with what I term 'soft' tension.

Soft tension is the feeling you get when you wake up in the morning and try to touch your toes and can get barely past your knees. You are aware that this isn't the permanent limit of your flexibility, and with a few warming-up movements and some gentle stretching you can regain and reach your true limit – however far down that may be.

True flexibility is limited by 'hard' tension. The hard tension marks the extreme limits of your movements, but it can and will be gradually softened by regular stretching.

Your aim is to turn hard tension into soft tension into no tension.

It is important to understand the concept of soft tension as it marks a boundary between your current range of movement and your true range of movement. This means that when you do a stretching exercise and meet resistance it is likely that this is temporary, soft resistance. With a little effort – and using an efficient technique – you can go through this to find the barriers of your hard tension.

Many people get discouraged when stretching as they discover how small their range of movement is in different joints. However, it may well be that the resistance they come to is just soft tension which, with just a little persistence, can be pushed back.

As you move a joint towards the end of its range of movement, resistance starts to build up. If you move quickly into any extended position, then the muscles will contract to prevent the joint from being injured. This is soft tension, and this can quickly harden if the body feels the joint is at serious risk of injury. This is why it is best to warm up before stretching. Your aim is to prevent the tension from hardening and limiting your range of movement. Another way to do tension building up during stretching is not to move quickly towards the limits of your range of movement. A slower movement will not trigger so much protective tension and you can move further into it.

Passive and dynamic stretching

There are two types of stretches – passive and dynamic.

Passive stretches use gravity to move you into the stretched position and enable you to relax into a stretch. Dynamic stretches rely on your own muscles to push you into the stretched position. Both types of stretch have their uses.

You should practice passive stretches first to get a general release of tension in that area. Then try dynamic stretches to enable you to move your limbs into that position through your own efforts. Bending forward to touch your toes is a passive stretch as gravity helps you on the way down. By contrast, sitting on the floor with your legs in front of you and reaching forward is a more difficult, dynamic stretch. You have only your core muscles to push you forward and oppose the resistance in your back and hamstrings.

Each of us is unique in every way. Your genetic makeup, the way you've lived your life, the habitual way you deal with stress mean that you have your own unique patterns of tension in your muscles. Hence there is no use in comparing yourself, flexibility wise, to another person because no direct comparisons can be made.

Take me as an example. I have relatively short legs and long arms, so it should be much easier for me to be able to touch my toes than someone with long legs and shorter arms. But that was something I couldn't get anywhere near all through my school years until I took up kung fu shortly after leaving school, and regular practice finally made it possible.

I often tell my students to ignore what others are doing during stretches and focus on themselves.

You are your only competition. Are you more flexible in this stretch than you were a couple of weeks ago?

Everyone will find certain stretches easy and others very hard. Obviously, it's of limited use practising the easy ones. It is the hard stretches that point to where your tension patterns are and so those are where you should be focusing your energy and time.

The rewards of increased flexibility are so great that it's well worth spending a bit of time once or twice a day to improve it. You should also try to vary not just which stretches you do but also how you do them, otherwise your routines will become just that: routine. So, wake up a little earlier tomorrow, get out of bed and do some stretches. I do them every morning when I get up. Treat yourself to a day that starts off with a body relatively free of tension and you will soon see what difference it can make to your life. If you have trouble sleeping then stretch before you get into bed and you will relax much easier into sleep.

There are hundreds of different stretching exercises in the world. Yoga alone has several hundred of them. It doesn't matter hugely which exercises you do. You will find ones that suit you and that you find enjoyable. Obviously, each joint needs to be stretched in different ways and there are several joints in the body all of which could be stretched in many different directions. Some exercises stretch more than one joint and these save time although you may find they are not as beneficial as stretches which focus on only one joint. This book doesn't aim to give you a range of stretching exercises - there are hundreds of other books or YouTube videos available that can do that. All I want to do is inspire you to make stretching an important part of your day. Having said that here are a couple of exercises that I find useful that gradually open up a range of joints and increase your mobility. They take only about five minutes and at the end you should feel significantly more relaxed and alive than you did at the start. You should do a lot more stretching than just these two but they will give you a good start.

The Hip and Shoulder Opener

1. Stand with your feet close together and your arms by your sides.

2. Raise your arms as high as is comfortable until you get to the edge of your soft tension. Don't force them higher. The first time you do this they may barely get above shoulder height.

3. Bend forward from the waist and, keeping your back straight as far down as you can, lower your arms then raise them up behind your back. Again keep within the level of soft tension. Lower your arms from behind your back then raise the arms and whole body upright again.

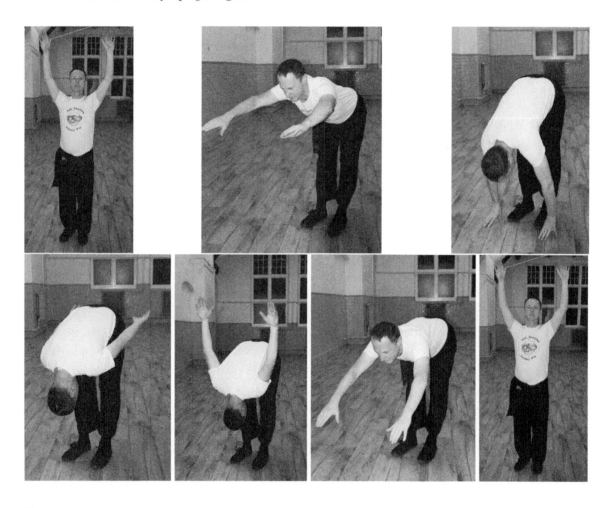

Repeat the exercise several times and you will find you can go a little further each time until you have gone through your soft tension to the limits of your hard tension. By this time your arms will be higher in the air and you will be able to bend further down. This exercise is great at mobilising the problem joints of the shoulders and hips. It gently stretches the hamstrings, back and chest muscles and strengthens the back. But, more than anything else, it makes you feel great - particularly when you're feeling tight and stressed. Do it several times a day.

The Clock

1. Stand with your feet wider than shoulder width apart with legs straight and raise your arms in the air.

2. Lean over to the left and gradually lower your body down towards your left foot then over to your right foot then back up to the vertical.

3. Repeat several times gradually extending your body further and further into the circle.

4. Then repeat moving down the right side and up the left side.

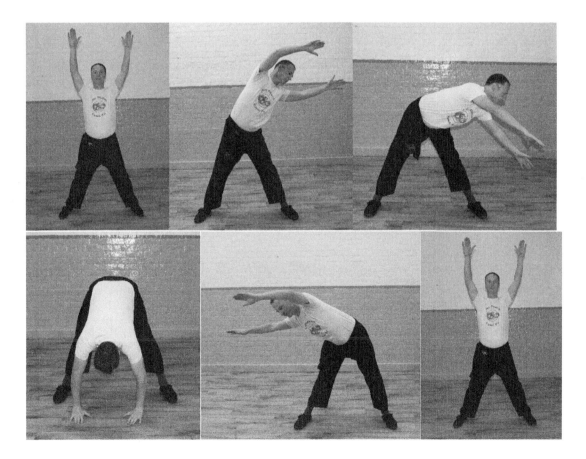

As with the previous exercise don't push yourself past your soft tension. Keep it comfortable all the way around and your range of movement will increase as you circle the body around. This is also great for the hips and strengthening the back. Do try to keep your back as straight as you can all the way through the exercise. A collapsed back is a weak back.

Circular Training

In kung fu we focus on learning to move the whole body in circular patterns. Why is this so important?

Circular movements are extremely good for the health of your muscles and skeleton. They open up the joints, promotes good circulation and releases a lot of tension in hard to stretch places.

A circular movement, when applied to an opponent is hard to resist as there is no set direction to which he can adapt. Even more difficult is a spiralling movement that is circling on more than one level. It is easy to take someone down if you are able to generate and connect circles in different joints of your body. Connecting them together builds up a wave of power that is almost impossible to resist.

Twisting and turning the body correctly means you must learn to move from your centre which is around the waist area. This maintains the mobility and function of the crucial central part of the body which is where we process our food (and, the Chinese believe, our emotions). Staying rooted to the ground, we twist the body and generate torque force to redirect an opponent's movements and force around us and sometimes redirect it back into them. Do not directly oppose an attack but merge with it and then circle it. In this manner, we maintain control and our opponent is forced into a circle that is hard for them to break out of.

Practice circling all your joints: ankles, knees, hips, waist, chest, shoulders, elbows, wrists and neck.

Circling these joints will do wonders for your tension levels and flexibility. Then, when you have gained a greater range of movement in the joints you should experiment with connecting the circles up. This is really good exercise and can have both a calming, almost hypnotic effect and an empowering one both at the same time. You will gain a lot more control over the joints in your body and will release many of the built-up tensions that you've stored there over the years.

One of the biggest problems with humans as they age is lack of joint mobility. Circling your joints is a wonderful exercise to keep them young and in good condition.

Try some of the following:

- Start by circling your wrists around then gradually work your way up to the elbows, include the shoulders, the chest, the neck and down to the centre and legs. Then circle the other way, again starting from the wrists.

- Alternatively start from the centre of the body. Move your waist around. Big circles is good for flexibility or smaller circles to build up a wave that will gradually move down your legs and up your spine to include your arms and head.

- Aim to get everything moving together and become connected. Go with the flow, don't force anything to move but let each joint join in as and when it wants to in the way it wants to. You will start to open up new neural movement pathways in your brain which will give you more and more control over your body.

- Become more experimental in the way you circle. Circling your arms over your head, for instance, is a good exercise.

Another key one we do in kung fu is to circle the centre by moving the weight onto one leg, lowering the stance, transferring the weight, raising the stance and transferring the weight again so the centre of the body is circling vertically. At the same time, it is twisting from side to side and these two movements generate powerful force in the middle of the body which can be connected to the arms for blocking, locking or striking.

Chapter 12.
Moving with Power

A MAP of your training

How do you learn a new physical skill? Within the vast realm of kung fu there are thousands of skills to learn and perfect. So much so that it would be impossible to learn them all even if you had several lifetimes to try. The task of learning any new skill is made even harder if you don't have a structure you can follow to enable you to learn the skill and be able to use it effectively. The structure that I teach is called MAP.

M is for Movement

The first step, of course, is to learn the basic movement. You learn the movement and through many thousands of repetitions you learn to do it more efficiently. The thousands of repetitions strengthen the muscles involved in doing the movement and by doing it to the point where it becomes tiring you also learn to relax the muscles that aren't involved.

All too often we use far more muscular tension in everything we do than we need to.

During our daily life, we often tense up muscles that have little or nothing to do with the task in hand. Learning not to trigger this tension conserves energy, gives you more control over the movement and doesn't cause tension in muscles that might resist the movement.

Most movements involve, or should involve your whole body. Every part of you should become involved to either move the body or to stabilise it against the forces that are acting or may soon be acting upon it. If you are doing a punch you're not just throwing your fist out. The movement should start from the ground with your back leg drilling into the ground to push your hip forward and the force goes up the back, through the shoulders and arms and out through the fist. At the point of impact, or expected impact you should be in perfect balance and in a stable position to minimise the return force. This is a large part of where the power comes from. It is important that all the force goes into moving your opponent and none of it comes back to move you.

So, the first stage is to practice the movement over and over again using your whole body as dictated by the movement. Only through endless repetition will you 'hardwire' the moves into your brain so that they become the way you habitually move when under duress.

A is for Application

Don't make the mistake of thinking each movement skill is teaching you a separate martial technique. It is way more than that. Each movement should be adapted so that it changes only slightly and can give you many different techniques. The yin circle for example could be a block followed by a strike, or a way of moving into a variety of wrist locks, an entry to a throw, a blocking of a kick followed by control of that leg through the knee joint and many other potential applications.

You learn to apply movement skills in stages. The first stage is against a non-moving partner who just holds out an arm or leg for you to block or manipulate. This teaches you correct positioning and distance skills. Only if your body is in the right position relative to your partner can the technique succeed. So, you apply the technique and strive to do so using as little effort as possible. This kind of demonstration is common on YouTube as it's easy to show how to defend against a non-moving 'opponent'.

Wherever possible you should try the technique out on as many different people as possible. This is perhaps the main reason why going to a class is essential if you want to learn any martial art properly. This is because everybody will react differently to your techniques so you need to learn to adapt them accordingly.

Once you can do the movement successfully on a non-moving partner then they can start to move, initially in a slow moving and predictable way but gradually they move faster and their attacks can become less predictable. Throughout this you need to continue to apply the principle of using as little effort as possible to make the movement work despite the increased pressure of the unpredictable attacks.

Eventually you will be able to apply the movement in many different ways against a wide variety of attacks.

P is for Power

When you can do the basic movement, and know some applications you need to start applying the principles that give the movement its power. Without power, you can learn a thousand techniques but they will be virtually worthless to you. However, once you learn to use real, whole-body power almost anything you do becomes a highly effective combat skill.

Real power doesn't come from big muscles. Real power comes from connecting your body together and rooting it firmly to the earth so that every move you make has the power of your whole body behind it.

Much of this book is about developing whole-body power and how to use it.

So first learn to do the Movement, then learn some Applications and finally develop the Power. In this way, when you practice with partners in class you are doing so without having yet learned and developed the full power to the movements. So, you are less likely to hurt or injure your classmates! This is the MAP to all good kung fu.

Moving your body

Before we look at how to move your physical structure let's start by looking at each part of it in turn and see how it fits together. Clearly it is only at the joints that we can move so we need to focus on those. Some joints will need to maintain stability while others move. Let's start at the top.

- Your head should be held erect and not be allowed to be pushed forward of the trunk. This bad habit comes from pushing the head forward to see screens better or while driving. It could be a symptom of vision problems. It leads to kyphosis, headaches and stress. The rest of the body should relax downwards from the head to maintain verticality.

- Your shoulders should be relaxed downwards in line with your chest, neither allowed to slump forwards or be pulled back. Dropped shoulders are important as they connect the arms firmly to the torso through the powerful action of the lat muscles.

- Your waist cannot move very much but the movements it makes are strong. The movement of the waist adds a lot of power to many kung fu skills so practice turning at the waist to strengthen the movement and enable a wider range of motion.

- Your hips can move much further than the waist but the movement isn't as strong. Learn to differentiate between turning the waist and turning the hips. When you need to turn the waist or hips, which will be in most of the moves then turn the waist first to get the power then add the hip movement to get extra range of motion. When standing in stances the hips should be tucked under slightly so that the tailbone is pointing downwards. This connects the legs to the torso.

- Your knees should never be locked straight and at least one knee should be bent at all times. Only a bent knee will strengthen your legs and let you use the power of those strong legs. You will never see a cat straighten its legs apart possibly for full extension in a jump. Then it will bend them again to absorb the impact force. Just like the cat, your leg muscles aren't just for moving but also act as shock absorbers to protect your joints from damage.

- Your feet should stay relaxed and not grip the floor.

- Your elbows are one of the most important joints for kung fu. To do backward and forward movements the elbows should be dropped downward. To do side to side movements the elbows should be raised to the horizontal. In this manner, the elbow always drives the hand forward, significantly adding to the power. There are many other aspects to good elbow use but these will be covered in future books.

Now that you know and hopefully have practiced the stances your legs will be getting stronger every day. Now it's time to learn how to use those strong legs to move your body in different directions and apply the force of the legs out through the arms. Here are a few of the stepping patterns we use.

Dragon Step

The dragon step is important in kung fu as it enables you to move forward against resistance. If someone is resisting and you need to move them backwards this is the way to do it. More importantly it develops the forward power for strong strikes. It teaches you to use your legs and keep the core strong.

How to do it

1. Stand in a dragon stance being aware of all the elements of the stance.

2. Keeping your front leg bent to the same degree bring your weight fully onto your front leg and pull your back foot in next to your front foot.

3. Now use the power of your standing leg to drive the other foot forward and slightly outward into a new dragon stance.

4. Make sure your body stays upright throughout the movement - there must be absolutely no forward or backward leaning.

When you have practiced this then it's important to do test it with a partner pushing against you. This is one move that definitely needs to be pressure tested. You should be able to move your partner backwards using the power of your legs and upright structure. Don't try to push with your arms. If you lean forward or backward you will lose the alignment and the power.

Half Dragon Step

The half dragon step is simple to perform but very useful for one reason. As I have mentioned before, when you are striking someone or otherwise applying force it is essential that you remain upright at the point of impact. Your body must be aligned with gravity so that the return force coming into you can be directed straight down into the ground. This adds immeasurably to your power and ensures that if you miss, or your strike is blocked, you are still in balance and able to adapt instantly.

However, if you are doing a forward strike and your opponent is slightly too far away for you to stay in balance the instinctive reaction of most people is for their body to follow the fist forward and to lean forward.

Leaning forward, even slightly, can be a fatal mistake and is the hallmark of an untrained fighter.

You should never lead your punches from the top anyway but drive them forward from your legs. The half dragon step gives you an extra foot or more of reach without having to lean forward and thus make yourself off balance.

To do it simply take an extra-long step forward into an extended dragon stance then instantly drag your back foot forward a foot or so to raise the stance again. Your upper body remains upright throughout. In this manner, your entire body weight is moving forward together whereas if you lean forward only the top half or less of your body weight is being used.

If you have to strike forward further than you can reach with your arms, spring forward off your back foot and drag your back leg up into a dragon stance. You will end up balanced and able to counter or follow-up as necessary.

Half Tiger Step

As with the half dragon step above this step simply involves taking a wider tiger stance then bringing your back leg closer and bringing your weight back onto it. This is good for moving closer to an opponent while maintaining a specific foot forward. There may be a reason why you want to keep your right or left foot forward and the half step enables you to do that and still stay mobile.

As you move forward using the half tiger step make sure that your body remains at the same height and doesn't bob up and down as you move. Maintaining the same height shows that you are driving the body forward correctly with the legs and the power is going forward and you remain rooted throughout. It is also useful to do the half tiger step backwards to increase the distance between your opponent and yourself where necessary. This step gives you a lot of mobility both forward and backwards while maintaining power.

Tiger to Dragon

Your stances give you strong legs and great power by making your body stable and compressed. However, it is usually when moving from one stance to another that powers techniques. The forward movement from tiger stance to dragon stance creates the forward power for a very strong strike. Similarly, the backward move from dragon stance to tiger stance will pull an attacker back and down and onto the floor quickly and smoothly.

The tiger to dragon transition is all in the legs and hips. In the tiger stance, your weight is mostly on the back leg so to move forward into a dragon stance you push your weight forward and at the same time turn your hips so they are square to your front foot. You need to reposition your back foot in a small arc going out and forward so that it goes from being ninety degrees out to the side to mostly pointing forward and you end up in a proper dragon stance with a gap between your legs to give you side to side stability. The turning of the hips should quickly guide your back foot into the right position.

To move back from dragon to tiger stance reverse the process. Step further back with your back foot and turn it out ninety degrees then bring most of your weight back onto it. It should go without saying by now that you need to keep your upper body vertical and not be tempted to lean back. Let your legs do the work and your entire body weight will come to bear on your opponent's arm so they will go down easily.

Always let your legs carry your upper body and everything will become easier.

Cat to Dragon

To move forward from a cat stance to a dragon stance, you simply move your front foot forward and slightly outward and bring your weight onto it. It is common for beginners to lift their weight as they are transferring it but you need to keep your weight down into the stance throughout the movement. The moment you lift your weight you lose your power and stability. The same goes for when you are pulling back into cat stance from dragon. Just bring all your weight back onto the back foot. You will need to slide your front foot back so that no weight is resting on it.

Cat Step

I love the cat step and could write a whole chapter on this movement alone. Within the Jade Dragon system as with several other good kung fu styles the cat step is used extensively, indeed in the advanced levels of some styles you may use little else.

The cat step involves stepping forward from one cat stance to another. The steps are fairly small - any wider and you would put weight on the front foot. Once you are within combat distance of an attacker you only need small steps to move around within the combat area. The weight is kept off the front foot so that it can quickly change direction and all the weight is rooted into the back foot. This root makes the cat stance more stable than you might think. Certainly, it is stable enough to be able to punch forward with power without being knocked backwards, once you have practiced and developed it properly. An assailant can't pull you forward as they would be pulling you onto your front foot and the stance is strong enough to resist quite a lot of pushing. If the push was too strong and you were going to fall backwards your unweighted front foot can easily step back into a dragon, cat or tiger stance to keep you upright and balanced.

The cat step is partly named as you are moving from one cat stance to another but it also helps you move like a cat - with stealth and balanced poise. It is the quietest of steps as you don't commit your weight onto your front foot until it has felt the ground first and is sure of its footing. This also helps prevent you from having to look down at your feet which tends to make you lean forward and then you lose alignment and balance.

To explain why this is important I should first explain how the average person walks. People do tend to walk in a number of styles however the following is the most common. Your average man or woman brings his weight slightly in front of his forward foot then swings his back foot forward and lets his weight drop onto it.

Stand up now, take a few steps and analyse the way you walk.

Humans are the only animal that stand and walk in the way we do. We don't have the luxury or stability of four legs but what we lack in stability we make up for in mobility and the use of our front limbs for carrying and manipulating objects.

Four-legged animals use their constantly bent rear-most leg to push their body forward using strong leg muscles. Us humans probably used to do that but now we are more likely to use gravity instead of leg muscles by leaning forward slightly and falling onto our forward leg. This isn't possible for four-legged animals as their other three legs keep them stable enough not to fall forward. Our habit of leaning forward contributes to the misuse of our body and means, as we age, that we are likely to end up stooped forward and in pain with limited mobility.

The cat step teaches us to stay upright and to use our legs properly. The front, unweighted foot feels the ground in front of us and the rear leg pushes us forward in a powerful and efficient way. We learn not to lean forward and to use our legs and hips properly, i.e. the way they have evolved to be used.

The cat step is very beneficial for your health as well as your kung fu.

How to do it

1. From a cat stance, you just toe your front foot out slightly.

2. Bring all your weight onto it and extend your back foot forward.

3. Now place it down on the floor without putting any weight onto it.

Points to remember

- As you are stepping forward stay upright and make sure you keep your hips tucked under slightly so that you don't lose power in your upper body.

- Don't look down as you step, use your foot to feel the ground before you commit your weight to it.

In combat you can't afford to look down at the floor you must be aware and alive to what is going on around you. The cat step teaches you to feel the ground with your feet so that you don't trip over tree roots, chair legs or the bodies of your previous victims! Another good point is that by keeping part of your attention on the ground under your feet it helps prevent you from panicking. I will explain more about how it does this in Part Three.

The cat step also allows for quick changes of direction. If your weight is on your left foot and you have your right foot forward you can turn right by turning your front foot out more and swivelling as you bring your weight onto it. Or you could turn left by turning your front foot inward. If you want to turn one hundred and eighty degrees you simply turn your front foot in by ninety degrees, bring your weight onto it and turn the other foot out. This move is fast and enables you to cover potential attacks from behind. This ability to toe in or out while in the cat stance is of vital use in getting you in the right position quickly. It is also used to change the distance of low kicks. Toeing in means your kicks have more reach (as it moves that hip forwards) whereas toeing out means you can kick someone while you are too close for normal kicks simply by toeing out and bring your leg up sharply onto their shin or knee.

Practice the cat step until it is smooth and easy. Practice changing direction with it, in fact you could just walk around your house a few times a day using the cat step. When you are familiar with it and well balanced try it with your eyes closed. This will force you to feel the ground and sharpen up your balance and other senses at the same time.

Chapter 13.
Guarding and Blocking

The extended guard.

In fight after fight after fight, in all styles of martial arts and mixed martial arts, I see men losing because they have a weak or non-existent guard.

It is becoming more and more common these days to see the boxing type guard being used in many martial arts and combat sports. This is assuming they use a guard at all. In so many combat matches I see guys with both hands down near their hips then, a second later, wondering how they got hit. Although it is useful in protecting the head and upper body from punches and high kicks the boxers guard does have its limitations.

- It's a purely defensive reaction, allowing your opponent to continue to attack at will.

- It places the arms in a structurally weak position.

- It wastes energy through retracting and extending the arms

There is another way, a better way. A way that has been handed down to us from the kung fu schools of old. That is to use your arms not to protect your upper body but instead to control the space between you and your opponent. This is the way used by many martial arts of old and everyone I have taught it to says it is more effective than the more common boxers guard. I call it the extended guard or the shield.

The practice is simple. You extend your arms forward towards your opponent so that they are in his space. Keep the arms slightly bent at the elbows and maintain the unbendable arm principle. One arm is up with the hand around face height while the other hand is lower down, a little above waist height. By

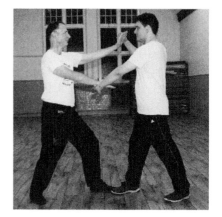

The extended guard

keeping one arm up and the other down you can easily protect yourself from both high and low attacks. By extending your arms into your opponent's space you are able to cover, anticipate and block or redirect attacks almost before he's even thought of using them.

It is surprisingly hard to get an effective attack past a good extended guard.

This guard position leaves your opponent with few options for attack. By limiting your opponent's attacking options, you can predict quite easily how he will react and already have your defences prepared. A simple turn of the waist will move your upper arm across your body to block on the other side or raising the lower arm and lowering the upper arm while turning gives a wide range of attack and defence options and are, in fact, the key moves in generating the yin circle and yang circle.

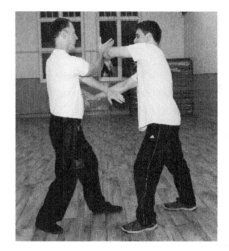

Generally, when using the extended guard for real your extended arms are covering your opponent's arms, your left to his right and vice versa. Your extended arms mean you can cover his attacks as soon as they've been launched and redirect them long before they reach their target. This is something I do with new students soon after they join to show them how effective this type of defence can be. I pit them against older and faster students and, as long as they keep their nerve and their shield up, the older students very rarely get anywhere near hitting with an effective strike.

Controlling opponent's arms with the extended guard

The shield does have to be strong and it gets its strength from a good physical structure. The most important thing is to keep the shoulders relaxed downwards. Most problems people have with extended guard is because they let their shoulders lift up. I see this time and time again in my classes and watching combat sports. It is essential that you learn to raise and lower your arms without raising your shoulders. This keeps your arms firmly connected to your trunk and makes your shield an integral part of your whole structure. If you are nervous and panicky then it's natural that your shoulders will rise. You must learn to become aware of it so that you can keep them relaxed down.

The shield is easy to learn and provides a more effective defence against kicks and punches than your typical boxers guard. It can literally be a lifesaver. So, lose your habitual boxers guard and learn to control the space in front of you. Many of the skills you'll learn in this and future books expand on this principle.

Yin and Yang Blocks

One of people's biggest fears is getting hit. I can understand that. It can involve blood, broken teeth, and lots of pain. One of the most important things to learn is how not to get hit. Most fights, particularly those involving untrained people involve punches or kicks. Many fights may involve some grappling as well but an effective block can help here as well by preventing the assailant from getting hold of you.

There are four basic blocks in the Jade Dragon system but as you progress you will learn many variations of these - indeed some variations will be introduced in this chapter. The four are the upper and lower yang block and the upper and lower yin block.

An upper block is blocking an attack in the upper part of the body ie chest to head area. A lower block is blocking an attack to the centre of the body ie hips and abdomen. Attacks to the legs can sometimes be blocked using a low block but more often than not is better simply to move your legs out of the way of them. For a block to be strong your blocking arm should be connected to and moving with your hips and legs.

A yang block is one that is moving from the centre of the body outwards while a yin block moves from outside to the centre of the body.

Upper Yang Block

The upper yang block is the most effective defence against the most common kind of strike - the punch that is swung to the head.

To perform the upper yang block, hold your arm out in front of your chest with your elbow pointing down and your hand palm up or facing you. Keep the arm almost straight with just a slight bend at the elbow and keep it as relaxed as possible. The amount of bend at the elbow doesn't change throughout the movement. For it to be fully effective you should learn the unbendable arm principle which will be covered shortly. Move your arm from the centre of your chest outwards to just past your shoulder. As you do this raise your elbow and naturally your hand will turn palm down. As you raise the elbow to the side take care not to raise your shoulder as well.

This, of course is only half the movement. You have to get your arm from where it currently is (usually down by your side) to that position in front of your chest. Generally, you just move it in an arc forward and in palm up and then sweep it out to the

side turning it palm down. Keep your arm feeling loose and heavy during the movement. Remember don't use too much force, or in-
deed any force or you will be fighting yourself rather than performing an efficient and effective
block. Practice it on both sides regularly until it
is a habit and one you can do instinctively if
needed.

Once you have got the arm movement down
then connect it to your hips and legs. Keep both
knees bent with your weight dropping down
through your feet and turn from the waist. Let
this turning movement move your arm across instead of using your shoulder muscles to move the
arm across. In this way, you are using a far
greater muscle mass and so the movement is far
stronger yet will feel more effortless to you. Again,
practice this on both sides until the movement is
hardwired into your body and brain.

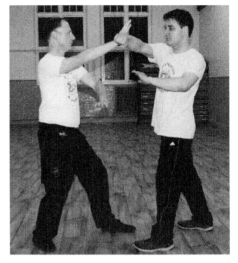

Yang block of opponent's punch

Lower Yang Block

This is performed in exactly the same way as the upper yang block but is not such an
important block although it can be useful against kicks. The initial position is the same
but your arm will swing down across the stomach area again with the elbow dropping
down and the palm facing down. Imagine someone punching you in the stomach and
you sweeping their punch down and out to the side. Let your arm fall downwards instead of pushing it down. Crazy as it may seem this
is far more effective. You can try it on yourself if
you don't believe me. Either push one arm down
onto the other or let the arm fall down and see
which is more effective.

Upper Yin Block

If you are being grabbed or punched directly forward then this block is your best bet. Raise your
hand palm up or facing you and with your elbow
relaxed down and sweep it across the front of your
body. This can be done quickly and it uses the
blade of your forearm (the little finger edge) as the
striking point.

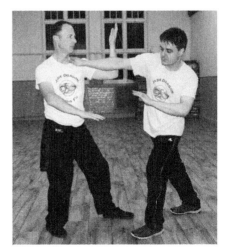

Yin block of opponent's grab

You can also block with the palm of the hand instead of the blade of the forearm. Obviously, the hand would be held palm inward with the fingers up instead of palm upward to do this.

Lower Yin Block

This isn't done in the same way as the upper yin block. The lower yin block is a very powerful block indeed. It's great against kicks and punches to the abdomen. To do it start with your arm hanging down then bring the elbow away from your body so that your forearm is still vertical then turn from the waist and bring the back of your forearm onto the target. The turning of the waist combines with the turning outward of the elbow to produce a stunningly powerful movement that will badly hurt any incoming leg or fist or anyone who tries to grab you around the waist. This is shown later in the book as a defence against grapplers.

Nobody likes getting hit so practice your blocks regularly. You need to find a partner to practice with. Start slowly. Start with predictable attacks then, gradually, increase speed and unpredictability.

Yang Circle

One of the first things my students learn is how to move their arms in circular patterns. The two main circles – the yin circle and yang circle are very important to learn. Practice them slowly and in fixed stances to start with and keep practicing them to strengthen them and make them more efficient. I still practice them regularly myself. For more information including training videos on them see the online section of our school website www.jadedragonschool.com.

Circular movements are better than linear ones for several reasons:

- A circle covers all angles so a circular block cannot easily miss

- A circle is a continuous movement. There is no stop and start so the power is constantly being expressed.

- Using a circular movement, you can merge with an incoming force and direct it into a different direction or back into the attacker. This is useful for many kinds of techniques

The yang circle is specifically developed to prevent an opponent from getting close to you. Rather than using a standard 'boxers' guard to protect the face and upper body the yang circle seeks not to protect your body but to control the space between you and your opponent. Throughout the yang circle both your arms are extended out into the space in front of you with just a small bend at the elbow. The arms move in overlapping circles moving up and across the body to around face height, then out just past the shoulders and down to waist height then in again. When one arm is up the other arm is down then they change places on either side. It makes good use of the outward yang force which maintains a protected zone of space in front of you. The yang circle is basically the same as the upper yang and lower yin blocks done continuously on each side. It can and should be practiced in all stances.

An unbendable arm, an unbreakable defence

I've just Googled "unbendable arm" and got about 7000 results. Almost every single one of the ones I read describes how to do it and either claims it to prove the existence of chi or, more commonly, to say that it doesn't prove anything of the sort. Virtually all of them dismiss it as a fun party trick and nothing more.

The unbendable arm is a concept that is seen primarily in tai chi and aikido. It is a way of holding your arm so that it cannot be bent at the elbow no matter how hard somebody tries. The best way to test it is to rest the back of your hand on someone's shoulder then get them to pull your arm downwards while you try to maintain a straight arm. Clearly if you are much stronger than them you can do this easily so find someone at least as strong as you are to test it on. When you resist in the normal way they should still be able to pull your arm down, bending it at the elbow and you fail.

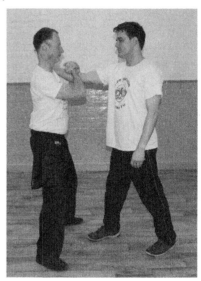

Testing the unbendable arm

To succeed at the unbendable arm, you need to learn to hold your arm a different way. Before your partner starts to push down, relax your arm and imagine a force going through the arm and being projected out through your fingers. Some people imagine a jet of water flowing out strongly and bursting through the wall/obstacles in front of them. Others imagine a beam of light projecting far out into the distance. Others find it better to imagine their arm as being twenty plus feet long. Experiment with different visualisations to see what works for you. The key thing is to maintain this mental focus of something going through the arm and increasing its apparent length and to stay as relaxed as you can while you do so. When you get this right, there is no way your partner, however strong he may be, can bend your arm. You must stay relaxed or it won't work. Any tension in your arm will have the effect of putting a block in the way of that flow of intention. It's like stepping on a hosepipe. Do so and the water just trickles out of the end.

The unbendable arm can be mastered in just a few minutes.

The unbendable am is quickly mastered so what is the point of learning it? Well in kung fu we use our unbendable arm a lot of the time. It is an essential element of the yang circle. By mentally extending through your arms as you circle them it makes them immeasurably stronger. The idea is to use your arms to prevent your opponent from entering the space in front of you with his arms, feet or body. Your unbendable arms, which are strongly connected to your waist and legs circle around and sweep his attacks out of the way. If your arms weren't unbendable when you blocked up and out there is a chance that your arm will bend at the elbow and the block won't be effective. This is particularly useful when facing an assailant with strong punching skills. The incoming punch should be stopped dead by your unbendable arm. If the arm bent it would only slow down the incoming punch which could then hit you anyway. If it is unbendable then it can seriously hurt anyone who gets blocked by it, particularly if they make contact with the blade of your forearm which, in a yang block, they would.

Back to the yang circle. In combat one of your primary aims should be to control your attacker and therefore control the situation. One way to do this is to grab them and manipulate their joints to gain compliance through pain. Unfortunately grabbing someone in the midst of combat isn't easy to do. This is where the circular element of the move comes in. When you block an attack, you continue to circle the arm or leg around thus maintaining contact with it for longer. This increases your chances of being able to grab the attacking arm or leg. While one arm blocks your attacker's arm and sweeps it across and down your other arm is already coming up to attack from the other direction. By learning this continuous circle of two arms you will never be blocking then hesitating, wondering what to do next. The next move will be microseconds behind the block putting you in a very advantageous position.

Training points

- Move your arms from the upper arm not from the elbow. The elbow joint should maintain the same angle - almost but not quite straight.

- Twist your upper arm so that the elbow drops and pulls in towards the centre of the body as it circles down and rises up so that the elbow is out as it circles up. This will also turn the palm from a yang position to a yin and vice versa.

- Move the arms as little as possible side to side. Use the legs and a turning of the waist to generate the sideways part of the circle.

- Do not lean forward at all as your arms lower or lean back as they raise.

Many of the skills you will find in this and future books use the yang circle. It is a key skill so practice it regularly. It will train your shoulders and develop fluid and efficient arm movements and the ability to express the power of your lower body through your arms.

Yin Circle

One of the major problems in all martial arts that involve grappling lies in how to get close to your opponent. Even a relatively unskilled person can use their arms to keep an assailant at bay so getting close to them to apply close-in techniques is often a big issue. Grapplers tend to get around this by going in low, under their arms and using that low stance as leverage to take them to the ground. But this low stance makes it difficult to see and react to attacks coming from different directions. It also exposes the sides and back of the head and upper back to attack and these are vulnerable areas which is why they are protected by rules in all grappling sports including MMA. In grappling competitions both fighters lean in and hold each other in the clinch before the action starts. Clearly this doesn't happen in real life. Luckily, there is another way, we call it the yin circle.

The yin circle is a vital skill to learn as there are many applications hidden within it such as strikes to the face, elbow locks and throws. Also, it keeps all the joints of the arm and shoulder limber and develops free movement of the shoulder girdle,

The yin circle is the opposite of its brother the yang circle. The arms circle in the opposite direction with the right arm moving anti-clockwise and the left arm clockwise. As with the yang circle when one arm is up, the other is down and they change places at the sides. The arms move down the centre of the body and up the outside. Unlike the yang circle there is some give in the elbow joint; indeed, it is this give that enables you to move in quickly close to your attacker. It does this by enabling you to bend at the elbow as soon as your arm blocks an incoming attack. The arm is nearly straight as it blocks then bends at the elbow as you move forward. This means you can continue to cover their attacking arm as you move in close for a lock or throw.

As with the yang circle you need to generate the arm movement through the legs and centre first and move from the upper arm so as to use the larger muscles of the body. As with all your skills you should practice it on its own for a while before trying it with a partner.

The yin circle uses yin force. It drops your opponent's force towards the ground and brings them in close to you. It enables you to counter-attack instantly and continuously. It is a key move in learning to throw effectively and is also the single best defence against high kicks, but more on that later.

Practice it well and the skills to come will become so much easier from your mastery of this fundamental movement.

Chapter 14.
Whole-Body Punching

The mechanics of punching

Most combat sports and martial arts use punches but they don't always fully understand how to get the best out of this useful weapon in their armoury. Read on to discover the biomechanics of the punch and find out how, with a few small changes you can dramatically and instantly increase the impact power of your punch.

There are many kinds of punches the most well-known being the ones that come from the field of boxing: the jab, the hook and the uppercut are good examples. Different punches come from different directions and are produced in different ways using different muscles. Most beginners punch very inefficiently. They are slow, lack power and end up off balance and vulnerable to counter attacks.

What is a Good Punch?

A good punch has the following characteristics:

- The body is rooted at the point of impact.

- There is no excess tension anywhere in the hand, arm or body which could slow down or weaken the punch.

- The punch finishes in a balanced and rooted position.

- The fist is formed correctly.

The above points apply equally to all punches. However, here we will also differentiate between punches that are done with power as opposed to punches that are done with speed.

To attain speed you must sacrifice power, to attain true power you must sacrifice speed.

Your fastest punch will never be your most powerful just as your most powerful punch will never be your fastest. It is easier to punch with speed than with power. Punching with real speed merely involves releasing as much tension as possible as any excess tension holds you back and slows you down.

Many people assume that to punch with power they need to build up their muscles with a lot of weight training. Let me make it clear now that although weight training does have its uses in physical development it has no role to play in punching power. In fact, there is a good chance that it will actually make your punches weaker.

I'm afraid it's true. When you are weight training you are using exercises that develop each part of your body at a time. You learn to isolate and disconnect each part of the body separately to train it. This is the opposite of what good punching requires.

To punch with real power, you need to coordinate your whole body together. In this way your legs, hips, waist, back, chest, shoulders and arms are all working as a team. They become, in effect, one large muscle and that one large connected muscle will always be stronger than the man who over develops specific muscles but can't connect them together to punch properly.

Weight training also strengthens the muscles that oppose the direction of the punch, particularly the biceps, so unless you have specifically trained to relax those muscles your weights will put the brakes on your punching power.

One of the most crucial elements that enables both power and speed is balance. You need to be balanced throughout the movement from the starting position to the end of the follow through.

Only when you are balanced are you in full control of your body. Any time you are out of balance, even slightly then tension will occur to prevent you from falling over. This tension is not under your conscious control so you have no idea which muscles will tense up or how much they will tense. This automatic tension that happens when you are out of balance will certainly prevent full and efficient movement of any kind.

Any movement you do while out of balance will be a compromise between what you want to do and what your body needs to do to bring you back into balance and prevent a fall.

A common beginners mistake is to clench the fist as tightly as possible when striking. When you clench your fist tightly it causes tension that goes up your arm into your shoulder, across your chest and so on. Try it now. Clench your fist really hard and you will feel how the muscles of your arm, shoulder and chest tighten. All this tension will act as a big brake on your punch making it slow, weak, and cumbersome.

Relaxed power is the key to a good punch. To form an effective fist simply close your fingers in loosely towards your palm and place your thumb between the first and second knuckles of your index finger. If you place your fist up to your eye you should be able to see right through it. You may think this fist would collapse and break on impact but you'd be wrong. It is a structurally sound fist. Try it and see. Hit yourself a few times with a tightly closed fist then with the one I've described above and feel the difference. I always encourage experimentation. Don't take what I or anyone else tells you on face value. Experiment for yourself and find out what really works.

A final word on fist formation - make sure the back of your hand and your forearm are in line with each other. If they aren't the force of the punch will go into your wrist and can easily damage it.

Start at The End

When beginners first learn to punch, it is common that their punches are quite wild and their upper body follows the fist forward towards the target. At the same time, their feet are uncontrolled and they can end up with one leg in the air or on tiptoe. This means they end up leaning forward towards their target and are off balance.

Part of the reason for this is that the arm is attached to the torso near the top so it's too easy to bend forward from the waist and follow your fist forward. This is why, in kung fu we always say to move from the centre of the body instead of the top. To prevent over reaching while punching I always get my students to start from the position they're going to end up in and work backwards from there. They practice standing in that final posture with fist extended. That way they are moving towards a balanced and familiar posture and aren't tempted to keep moving beyond it.

A good example of a power punch is the dragon punch which we'll cover in a moment. This punch ends up in the dragon stance so you practice by starting off in this stance then pull back slightly with your torso and punching arm then move forward back to that dragon stance with extended arm. Keep doing this gradually pulling back further until you can punch into that dragon stance without over-reaching. You can do the same with many other skills. Start at the point where force will be applied and make sure you are balanced and stable at that point and then get used to moving into that position.

Power comes from using your legs and waist to drive your body through the movement and to end up in a balanced and stable position

Coordinate Your Body

When practicing any technique try to feel which parts of your body are moving together and coordinate them as closely as you can. With most punches, the back knee and the elbow of the punching arm work together. They both bend together and straighten together. When one of them is fully straight the other should also be fully straight and you should stop moving. To try to move beyond this point would mean you're leaning forward which makes you vulnerable.

There are two classic t'ai chi chuan sayings which are of great help here:

"The feet move with the hands, the elbows move with the knees and the shoulders move with the hips."

"When one part moves, all parts move and when one part stops, all parts stop."

In any movement try to feel how the parts of your body work together, then move everything together and focus on keeping all parts coordinated.

Maintaining a good root at the point of impact is the most important point of gaining a powerful punch. When you make contact with an opponent a force will build up between your fist and the target. That force has to go somewhere and it will take the path of least resistance. If your opponent isn't rooted and you are the force will go into his muscles and push him backward whereas in you the force will go through you and down into the ground. In my experience and testing on hundreds of students the power of a good punch is around 30% muscle strength and 70% proper alignments and stability)

I can throw around and punch down men who have twice my muscle mass with very little effort because I know how to align my body correctly to the forces at play and they usually don't. So, practice your stances and learn to move with relaxed power.

One final word on punching power. I mentioned in the introduction that I learned how to use the power of the mind to add power to your movements. There is a simple mental technique you can perform that will add significant power to your strikes.

When an average person punches, they tend to focus on the punching hand and pushing it as fast and hard as possible into its target. This is inefficient as it tends to tense the bicep muscle which will tighten and oppose the movement. It is better to focus on your elbow instead of fist when punching.

Try this now. Punch a few times while focusing on your fist then try a few times focusing on your elbow instead. When focusing on the elbow your hand will fly forward with far less effort. It won't feel as powerful to you but that is because you are less tense in the arm. It will feel significantly more powerful to your opponent and, again, you can try this for yourself. Stand in front of a wall and push into the wall with your hand. Your body will move back because the wall is more stable then you are. Now try pushing into the wall while focusing on your elbow. Your body will go back much further. This shows how much more forward force there is when you focus on your elbow instead of your hand. There are many more ways of using the mind to affect the way the body is used and how much power different movements can have. I will go into some more in later books.

The dangers of hand conditioning

Ever since we first learned to stand and walk on two legs humans have used their hands to reach out and connect with the world. Our hands are highly sensitive and very dexterous and it's important that we look after them. Too many martial artists end up in their old age with hands that can hardly move and that lack the power and finger dexterity of their youth. They do this through unbalanced and reckless hand conditioning training.

'Boards don't fight back'

The above quote is a classic line from Bruce Lee's film 'Enter the Dragon' but it's as true today as it was then. A lot of people spend a lot of time developing the ability to break inanimate objects. But this skill, impressive as it may look, has little to do with actual combat. It's more in the line of a circus trick that is often used as good marketing for the school.

The most important reason to avoid power breaking practices is the short and long term damage to the hands and wrists or whatever else you may be tempted to try and hit solid objects with. Bone deformations, callouses, hairline fractures, arthritis and so on are common among those who are tempted to try breaking practices. Any practice that has little functional value yet can damage your body severely should have no place in your training schedule. Indeed, good kung fu schools believe that any practice that damages the body has no place in training. It is illogical to engage in a practice that leaves your body damaged and in a worse state to defend yourself than before you started.

So, what is this training for? Supposedly it is to develop a 'killer strike' that will stop the fight dead. But suppose you were to use your 'killer strike' in real combat. One of two things would happen. Either it would be blocked or would miss its target - all that training wasted, or worse it could hit its target and do far more damage than you intended as you have never hit a person with this force before. The genuine risk is that if your big power strike was used successfully in actual combat it could seriously injure or even kill someone (and yes this has happened). Power breakers aren't used to slowing down or controlling the force of their strike - they need maximum speed on impact to smash boards or bricks. This lack of control goes against the philosophy of most respected martial arts. People are also not built like boards or bricks anyway - we are essentially big bags of water and behave like it when struck hard. The training is both dangerous and unrealistic.

For martial artists who shun power breaking you need to increase both the sensitivity and the power of your hands. Of these two qualities sensitivity is the most important. Hands only need to be powerful when you want to grip your opponent with force. However, they do need to be able to transfer the force coming through the rest of the body and arm through the hand and into the opponent without damaging them.

Iron palm training

Iron palm training is the description for various methods for training the hands to be able to withstand striking forces. When done properly and with the use of the correct herbs etc. it will make your hands strong without loss of sensitivity or damage. Different schools have developed different methods of iron palm but there are two main versions and you can use either or both.

External iron palm.

The external way involves gradually striking your hand into more and more solid surfaces eg sand, gravel etc. When done badly you are likely to cause harm to your hands and lose dexterity and sensitivity as well as causing you unremitting pain. External iron palm training aims to turn your hand into a hammer that will absorb much of the impact force itself and many believe that without this conditioning training your hand would break.

To make iron palm effective it must be trained gradually.

If you rush any form of iron palm training you can destroy the nerve endings and put intolerable strains on the bones and soft tissues of the hand or body. This nerve damage will severely reduce the sensitivity in your hands which will affect your reflexes and ability to react quickly to what you can see and touch.

There are herbs available to help the hand recover between practices, particularly the legendary dit da jow. However, unless you are a herbalist yourself you won't know what's been put into this and there is a lot of fake dit da jow being sold for high prices which is of little, if any, use.

Internal iron palm

Internal iron palm involves contracting the breath into the palm to achieve the same effect but without loss of sensitivity or incurring such damage to the palms. It takes a lot longer, some say around 3 times as long to get the same effect. Also, it is important that you have been taught good basic breathing practices first. This is beyond the scope of this book but part of the training process will be included in the third book of the series.

Internal iron palm can be mixed with external to speed up the process and lessen the damage. However, if you intend this type of training do be aware that both have serious risks attached and make sure that you find a Master who has undergone such training without severe damage to his hands.

While serious Iron Palm training is not recommended without qualified instruction there are some things you can do to strengthen your hands:

- Push ups can be done on the knuckles however, these must be done on a soft surface ie carpet or grass. No wooden or concrete floors which will damage the knuckles.

- Push ups can also be done on the fingertips or the backs of the hands. This is not as difficult as it sounds and can be done on any surface.

- Towel wringing - doesn't have to be a towel, a tshirt or other cloth will do just as well. Twist it as if you were wringing water out of it. Then change direction ie left hand up instead of down. This is great for all forearm muscles and grip strength.

Weapons training

Any kind of weapons training will help develop your hands and grip strength. This, in fact, is the preferred way in many martial arts. The weapons teach you to remain relaxed and sensitive in the hands for moving the weapon yet be able to grip hard when necessary to produce the whip-like force through the body and into the weapon that higher levels of weapons training require.

In many traditional schools, weapons are still a key part of training. Apart from their obvious use in defence they also help develop the student properly for hand to hand combat. The advantages included:

- Regular practice increases the strength and flexibility of the hands, wrists and forearms.

- They teach the practitioner how to manipulate the weapon efficiently, when to grip hard, when to let go, when to apply force and when not to. The use of the weapon closely mirrors the use of the hands in actual combat.

- The hands have to be sensitive to the feel of the way the weapon is moving and be able to transmit power out to the end of the weapon.

- Two handed weapons, particularly the staff, teaches students to use their hands together to support each other.

- Regular training helps prevent the common beginners mistake of gripping too hard and not being able to unfreeze that grip. This could be dangerous in combat if you weren't able to let go of your attacker to block or counter attack. Regular weapons training loosens the grip without sacrificing power and teaches you to grab and let go at will.

The use of weapons also helps to focus the power along the weapon to the tip. This trains the practitioner to focus their locks into the arms of an opponent to take control of an elbow or shoulder with virtually no effort. Proper use and positioning of the hands makes this highly effective.

Sensitivity training

Hands tend to hold onto a lot of tension so it's also important to learn to keep them loose and relaxed. Remember - the more relaxed they are the more sensitive they are which helps develop lightning reflexes. This means that they will feel the movements of your opponent quickly and accurately so that you can adapt and respond appropriately. Too much tension will prevent you from getting good feedback or from being able to react in time. Sensitivity comes through relaxation. You can gain sensitivity in your hands simply by giving them your attention.

1. Focus your attention on the tips of your fingers. Feel them start to tingle.

2. Brush your fingers and hands lightly over different surfaces and see how much feedback you can get both with eyes open and closed.

3. Close your eyes and explore the immediate surroundings with your hands. Only by repeatedly bringing your attention into your hands can sensitivity be increased. Regular practice will sharpen your reflexes and deepen your awareness of your surroundings.

4. Learn to use only as much force as is necessary to manipulate the world around you. For example, learn to hold your knife and fork more lightly, as if they were very fragile. Don't grip your steering wheel hard but lightly and make the movements from the elbows rather than hands. This will also take some of the tension out of your shoulders.

Iron palm training can be useful if it is taught properly by a qualified person who still has full dexterity and sensitivity in his hands as well as iron like power.

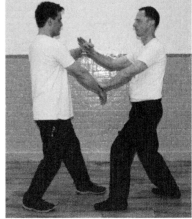

Traditionally hand sensitivity is increased by push hands type drills in class as well as the sensitivity training drills I mentioned above. Push hands training enables you to directly read and react to the movements of another person.

Look after your hands, develop their sensitivity and aliveness but also remember that they are at the end of a chain of muscles and joints and it's no good having strong yet sensitive hands if the rest of the body is locked with tension. However, release of tension in the hands will greatly aid relaxation in the arms and the

Push hands practice

shoulders. Practice touching and sensing and see just how relaxed, fast, and sensitive your hands can become. Then, when needed they can become weapons of steel before relaxing back into softness again.

Dragon Punch

The dragon punch is the basic punch that is done in the Jade Dragon kung fu system. It is a powerful forward strike, generally aimed at the chest area and the non-striking arm moves out at the same time to block or cover the striking arm. When practised this punch will take an assailant straight to the floor and wind him for seconds, even minutes. When developed fully it can break ribs easily yet takes almost no effort to perform. My students, even those with extensive prior martial arts experience, are always amazed at the power of this punch. When striking somebody holding a strike shield or pads this punch can easily make them fly backwards, even with little training.

The dragon punch is the most useful power strike in the Jade Dragon system. It uses correct biomechanics to ensure that your body is in the most stable and powerful position it can be when your fist makes contact with your opponent. This means that mastering the dragon punch enables you to punch very hard regardless of your size or how strong you are.

On top of this the dragon punch teaches you to use both arms together so that your non-punching arm is either blocking or supporting your punching arm. I know and teach literally hundreds of defences against punches. There are more potential defences than you probably even believe are possible. Yet 90% or more of those counters won't work against the dragon punch simply because the guard arm is there to counter those counters. Using the dragon punch makes sure that far more of your strikes will hit their target, and hit it hard.

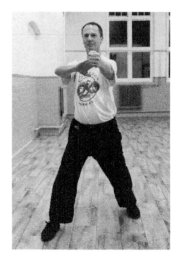

When learning and training the dragon punch always start by learning to stand in the final position. This is the position your body will be in when your fist hits its target. At this point your arms, legs and torso are strongly linked together to ensure you get maximum impact value and that you can handle the return force. Remember, for every action (or force) there is an equal and opposite reaction (or force).

Dragon punch final position

The final position is as follows:

1. Stand in the dragon stance. If you are punching with your right fist you are forward on the left leg and vice versa. With this type of punch, you always strike with the arm that is opposite your front foot.

2. Extend your striking arm forward so that that there is a slight bend at the elbow. Point the elbow downwards and keep it in front of your torso. This will naturally turn your striking hand slightly palm up but twist your wrist so that your fist is vertical. This is a little-known secret of effective forward strikes. This keeps your striking arm in a structurally strong position that can project and absorb force from the front with virtually no effort. As always if you doubt this then try it for yourself.

3. Extend both elbows forwards towards your opponent. This uses extra stabilising muscles and releases tension in the back of the shoulders so enabling the return force to flow through you and down into the ground. Again, this makes a big difference to the power and stability of both the strike and accompanying block.

Practice standing in this position and get someone to push into your extended fist or try pushing hard it into a wall until you can do so without moving your structure.

To perform the dragon punch step into a cat stance then drive your body forward into the dragon stance and, at the same time, strike forward with the opposite arm to your forward leg. You can step out in any direction so this punch can quickly be applied to an attack coming from any angle. Generally, if your opponent is coming from your left you would be stepping out with the left leg, blocking with your left arm and striking with your right arm whereas if they come from the right you step out with the right leg, block with the right arm and strike with the left arm. You need to be equally proficient on both sides.

Points to remember

*   Don't just step forward with your front foot but actively drive your body forward from the back foot. Your knees should be bent before you start as you cannot drive forward from a straight leg. This is why we move into a cat stance or tiger stance first. This driving forward action puts the weight of your whole body behind the strike.

*   Make sure as you drive forward that your front foot roots into the ground just before your fist hits its target otherwise you will lack power and stability on contact.

*   At the point of impact your striking arm should be almost straight at the elbow but not locked out. Don't focus on the chest of your opponent if that is your striking point. You need to focus through the striking point to the spine or even behind it.

- Your elbow should be pointing down with the fist in the vertical rather than horizontally aligned. If you were holding a stick in your hand it would be vertical rather than horizontal. There is no twisting movement in this punch. A twisting movement raises the elbow which tends to raise the shoulder which makes the arm movement less stable. If you doubt this then try it. Push against a wall with your elbow out to the side then try it again with the elbow down and feel which one pushes you back more. A straight forward punch with the elbow down (or twisted in towards the chest) is more powerful than one with the elbow out to the side. I know that many martial arts teach a forward strike where the fist twists to the horizontal position and the elbow comes out to the side but just because many others teach that way doesn't make it better. That position works well in other types of strike where the fist circles around to strike from the side but not so well with direct forward strikes. Try them both and feel which is more powerful. Keeping your elbow down also keeps it out of the way of your opponent's arms and makes for a much faster strike. From your arm hanging down by your side it takes only a fraction of a second to raise it slightly, bend the arm at the elbow and shoot it forward. There is no need to chamber the strike, this only slows it down and advertises what you're doing to your opponent.

- Your spare hand is important. Unlike in many martial arts we do not teach to leave it at the hip but to keep it extended out in front of the body where it can be used to cover and protect you. A spare hand at the hip is virtually useless. It's only purpose is to be driven forward as a strike but is easily spotted and blocked. It cannot protect you from the hip position. With the dragon punch the spare arm is extended in front of the body and bent at the elbow so that the fingers point towards the inside of the forearm of the striking arm. This position will of course change should the spare arm be required for blocking or covering a possible attack.

- Keep your back heel on the ground as you strike and your body upright - don't lean forward at all.

Tiger Punch

The tiger punch is another strong punch that can be applied at speed. It ends up in the tiger stance, hence the name. As you end up with most of your weight still on your back leg it is easy to drive forward from there into a follow up dragon punch.

The tiger punch is easy to do once you have mastered the tiger stance. Simply step forward with your right foot for a right punch and at the same time move your right arm forward to strike. Strongly resist the temptation to bring your weight forward for this strike. Your arm and foot should move forward together and your foot should hit the floor just before the fist makes contact so that you are rooted at the point of impact. The spare arm is held across the chest with the elbow bent no more than ninety degrees.

Points to remember:

- Your foot should land just before your fist.

- Drop your weight onto your back foot.

- Keep your spare arm across your chest bent no more than ninety degrees

- Keep your punching elbow pointed down.

Chain Punch

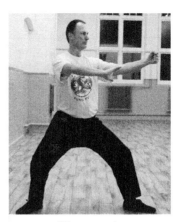

Tiger punch

Anyone who has watched any of the Ip Man films will be aware of the signature wing chun chain punch. Although the punch only travels a short distance it is delivered at high speed and several punches can be delivered in a single second.

This skill is by no means unique to wing chun nor is it likely that they developed it. Variations of this strike can be found in many styles of kung fu. Here I will teach the basic punch but there are a wide variety of different ways of using it and applying it. In fact, all the animal styles I practice and teach use it in a different way.

In all things kung fu there is a trade-off between speed and power. The faster a move is generally the less power there is behind it. Some martial artists train specific strikes or kicks to break solid objects. Apart from the inherent dangers in power breaking these types of strike require a period of time to build up the power. That power can't be released instantly as it would need to be in real combat so, although they can demonstrate that such a strike is possible they are of limited use in a real fight. Chain punches can be released instantly seemingly out of nowhere. They also don't require that you commit a lot of force to a single technique.

In kung fu you should never commit to a technique unless you are sure it will succeed.

The usual kung fu strategy is to use non-committing moves that test the opponents' alignments, balance, skill level and so on. When you find a weakness, and are in the right position to exploit it then you can commit to a technique but before that it is play time, keeping yourself safe and testing for your opponent's weak areas. This is where sparring training comes into its own.

The chain strike is an ideal example of this. Instead of relying on one big power strike the chain strike is a rapid-fire series of strikes aimed at overloading your opponent's defences. A fast chain strike attack is both physically and psychologically devastating. None of the strikes on their own are particularly powerful but they come in at between five to ten strikes per second depending on your skill level. Each strike can hit the same point or target different areas to further confuse and overwhelm your opponent.

When you strike an opponent in this manner It is easy to see how he is reacting to this kind of attack and to adapt your attack to different targets and different angles continuously. It is like the difference between firing a bullet from a gun and squirting water from a hose pipe. One is a single committed attack that can't be changed where the other is a continuous, changeable attack that can continue to target the opponent as he tries to escape it.

The chain strike is easy to learn but requires practice as it puts a lot of strain initially on the chest and front of shoulder muscles.

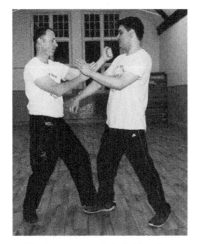 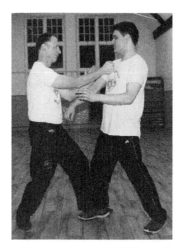

Chain punch – left fist leading   Chain punch – right fist leading

How to do it

1. Hold your arms in front of your body with your elbows close together and your palms facing each other. Keeping the elbows close together has two purposes. Firstly, it protects your centreline from being attacked. Secondly, it strengthens each of the strikes. Yes, it will feel unnatural and uncomfortable at first, but persevere, and it will become easier to do, stronger and, of course, faster. If your elbows are sliding back past your ribs then you're doing it wrong. The elbows should be kept in front of the chest so that if your hand comes back too far your upper arm will bump into your chest. Try it with a partner. Hold your arm with the elbow at the side of the chest, and then push them away. Then try pushing again, with your elbow in front of your chest. You will find the second move, to be significantly stronger, even though you didn't use any additional force. It is all to do with stability and alignment. So always keep your elbows close in, when doing chain strikes.

2. Extend one hand in front of the other and close the leading hand into a loose fist. The trailing hand should be close to the forearm of the leading hand with the fingers pointing to the wrist.

3. Lower the leading hand slightly, open the fist and draw it back while the rear hand moves forward and closes into a loose fist.

4. As always, stance is important. As you're striking forward you need one leg in front of the other with both knees bent for stability and most or all of the weight on the back leg. The cat stance or a shortened tiger stance are best for this type of strike.

5. Repeat the movement continuously.

Points to remember

• The chain punch is a fast, striking movement, where both hands are circling forward, the front hand is striking while the rear hand is covering.

• Keep the circles small to maintain the speed and focused power.

• Keep the elbows held close together, in front of the chest.

• Maintain a good stance. Cat stance is best.

The method I teach differs from the wing chun method as we teach you to open and close the hands coordinated with the forward and back movement of the arms. This enables the move to be adapted into a grabbing technique as well as a strike. With practice, you can grab an arm then quickly open your hand to let go of it then close your hand again to strike. All within a fraction of a second.

Remember that this is a punch, so don't just wave your arms in vague circles, but focus on striking an imaginary object in front of you.

Once you have developed some stamina, and fluidity in this move, then you can gradually speed it up, and learn to vary the angle of the strike.

Reverse Chain Punch

This is another difference from the wing chun method. With the reverse chain punch your arms circle backwards. So, as your leading hand strikes it moves slightly upward instead of down and the next hand comes forward from below. Otherwise the move is exactly the same.

If an opponent blocks your attacking arms down the forward chain strike can continue to attack over his downward block. But, if he blocks your arms upward it would foil a forward chain strike. This is where you would switch to a reverse chain punch which would attack under his rising block. Again, try it and see.

Chapter 15.
Kicking in Real Life

Don't kick high

It surprises many people to realise that a lot of kung fu schools, possibly even most of them, don't advocate high kicks. They are considered impractical and dangerous to the practitioner. The dangers usually outweigh the benefits unless you are protected by rules that don't allow your opponent to react in the ways that attackers in street encounters might.

High kicks require a high degree of flexibility, power and speed to get your leg from the floor up to your opponent's head before he can react. They also leave you standing on one leg so your balance is easily compromised and they expose vital areas to counter attack. In fact, there are really few upsides to high kicks apart from the fact that they look good, hence their prevalence in martial arts films. High kicks are what people see all the time in films and TV so they assume that this is what all martial artists do.

The Okinawans developed the skills to kick high and hard. They developed both standing and flying high kicks for the sole use of kicking mounted samurai off their horses. If you are on the back of a horse you have no way of avoiding such kicks. But, if you are standing on the ground you can avoid or block them far more easily.

It is more practical to kick low than high. Low kicks are hard to see coming, they are often too low to block with the arms and can be done quickly so that the attacking leg is back on the ground before an opponent can take advantage of the fact you're on one leg. They also don't expose your groin and other vital areas to attack.

Unless you are planning to train a combat sport or want to show off to your friends, don't spend too much time trying to train for high kicks. Yes, they develop strong and flexible legs and a strong core but they aren't realistically useful in street conflict. Most martial artists who specialise in high kicking say they do so because leg muscles are stronger than arm muscles. Therefore, kicks are more powerful than punches. It is certainly true that leg muscles are stronger than arm muscles there's no denying that. But the point is that when you punch properly you do not only use your arm muscles. A good punch uses the legs, hips, waist, back, chest, shoulders and arms together.
A proper punch is more controllable and less risky than any kick. Your feet stay on the floor so you can move around and maintain your balance and adapt far more quickly to what your opponent is doing.

The two most useful kicks for general self-defence are the low front kick and the back kick. The low front kick uses relaxed power and has the element of surprise as well. It can be a devastating kick when trained properly. The back kick is the strongest of the kicks as it uses the biggest muscles in the body. It is probably the only kick that can be used effectively above the waist as it is such a difficult kick to block. Train these regularly as they will become a part of your arsenal.

Front Kick

The front kick appears to be easy. You raise your knee then extend your foot towards your target. But don't forget your MAP. It is the power behind the kick that is important and that power comes from your rooted stability at the point of impact.

The Movement

1. To train the front kick you must learn to stand on one leg in the crane stance.

2. Once you can comfortably stand balanced in the crane stance for at least 30 seconds on each leg then practice raising and lowering your leg up into the stance, holding for a few seconds then lowering again. Do this slowly and under full control the same number of reps on each leg. Focus on keeping your weight relaxed down onto your standing leg. Make absolutely sure that your upper body doesn't sway back or forward as you raise and lower your leg. Also, don't raise your stance as you raise your leg, keep your supporting knee bent and relaxed downwards. Strong back muscles will keep your body upright and counter the weight of your leg when it's stuck out in front of your body.

3. Next raise the leg into the crane stance and extend at the knee again moving slowly and under full control back and forward. Then extend it at the knee, lower it straight legged, raise it straight legged again then bend the knee back to the crane stance and repeat on both sides. This training along with flexibility training on the hamstrings and hip flexors will develop your front kicking skills tremendously.

The Application

Although the above training will gradually enable you to get higher with your front kicks remember that this kick is primarily used for targets of waist height or below. This is not a high kick although the training will help in other ways. The front kick is most often used to kick into the opponent's knees, groin or stomach area. Because of the danger of the kick being blocked and the leg grabbed you must never leave the leg stuck out in front of you. Kick, then ground your leg again as quickly as possible.

It is important never to broadcast to your opponent your intentions. Therefore, you should practice kicking with no movement of your upper body. At first there is a tendency for the upper body to rock backwards and forwards and this clearly signals in incoming kick. Keep your weight over your standing leg and learn to kick from different stances without broadcasting them while still maintaining good balance.

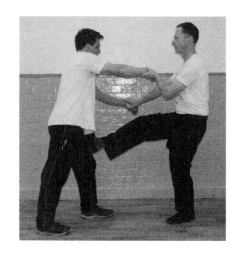

A key component of effective application is distance. Get the distance wrong and you'll either not have enough room to raise the leg for the kick or the opponent will be too far away to reach. Practice with a kick bag or just kicking a wall to get used to the distance needed to kick effectively. You can adapt the distance required for the front kick as follows:

If your opponent is a little too far away for a standard kick then turn your standing foot outwards and/or your kicking foot inwards. This will extend your hip on that side and give you a little more reach.

If the opponent is in too close for you to raise your leg then turn your kicking foot outwards. This will turn the knee and the hip out and enable you to raise it up sharply onto their shin or kneecap. There's no way they can see this kick coming. It is a more powerful kick than you'd think and a great technique for close in fighting.

The final thing to note about application is that this kick can be done to distract an opponent's attention downwards. If your opponent has a good defence then it is often worth a low kick to take their attention downwards. This divided attention will often weaken their upper guard and allow you to counterattack their upper body successfully.

The Power

As with the majority of our skills the power comes largely from your body's stability at the point of impact. This power comes from your root and to have a useful root you must be relaxed downwards with your supporting knee kept well bent. This is why the front kick is not a high kick. The moment you start kicking above the hips then your leg must be kicking upwards which will lift your root upwards and destabilise you. Only by kicking straight forwards or downwards can you maintain your root and your power. In many kicking sports, high kicks force the practitioner to come up onto their toes to deliver the kick but this leaves them in an unstable position and their balance is up for the taking.

To avoid this, you must train your stances, particularly the crane stance to the point where you can stand on one leg and push someone away from you without losing balance and falling over.

The front kick is usually done as a moving forward movement. It comes up quickly from a short dragon stance into the legs of the incoming opponent and after the kick you drop your leg down and bring your weight onto it. As such it is just like walking normally forward with a powerful, low kick as each foot steps forward. It was used to great effect in the film 'The Bourne Ultimatum' during the fight at Waterloo Station.

Practice your crane stance and leg raises and extensions and you will have a very powerful move to add to your growing arsenal.

Back Kick

The back kick and the front kick are the two main kicks taught to new students in the Jade Dragon School. The back kick is an important one to learn and practice as it can protect you against attacks from behind, it is very versatile in its use and is the strongest kick in our repertoire.

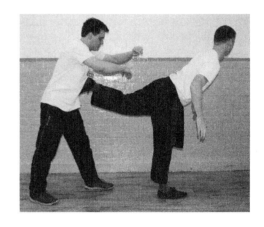

The back kick is so powerful because it uses the big muscles of the hamstrings, gluteals and back. For these big muscles to come into play the back kick must be a proper back kick with the hips held square to the front.

If the hips are allowed to turn, even a small amount to the side then it becomes more of a side kick and then it uses different, and much smaller muscles. This side kick is only a fraction as powerful as a true back kick.

The movement

1. To do a back kick stand in a dragon stance with your back to your target.

2. Push off your front foot to bring your weight over your back foot.

3. Keeping your hips facing the front, kick your lifted leg behind you with your toes pointing down. Then place it back down into another dragon stance.

Points to remember

*   Flex your kicking foot, don't point it, and keep your toes pointing down as much as possible.

- In order to see the target that you're kicking turn your head in the direction of your kicking foot i.e. turn your head to the right if kicking with the right leg. It is important that this turning of the head doesn't also turn your hips. Keep them square. You will be able to see your target in your peripheral vision.

- Straighten your kicking leg as much as you can. At least to start with this will be more difficult than it sounds.

- It is permissible to bend forward somewhat to increase the height of the kick.

- Train the movement slowly and in full balance. To start with you may use a wall or object to keep your balance but try not to rely on this and to get rid of is as soon as possible. It is good practice to be able to perform the kick in perfect balance and to be able to stop and hold the position at any point in the movement.

- As always, being rooted and balanced at the point of impact is crucial.

The application

Not only is the back kick a powerful one but it is difficult to defend against. It comes up out of nowhere and can project a man several feet backwards. The kick will always travel in the direction of the heel of your supporting foot.

With this in mind you can be quite creative in your use of this powerful kick. By turning your right foot to face the left you can turn your body towards the left and deliver a powerful back kick with your left leg towards your right or vice versa. Similarly, you could take a step towards an opponent with one foot but swivel on it so as to turn away from the opponent and deliver a back kick with the other foot. There are some joint locks where an opponent may twist your arm so that you have your back to him. You can use this technique well under these circumstances. Step forward with your foot as you turn your back then instantly kick back into his shins or knee.

The power

You should know by now that a major component of the power in all these skills is the ability to relax downwards into the ground at the point of impact. The back kick also gets its power by recruiting most of the large muscles in the body. As the kicking leg moves back into its target both legs straighten somewhat, the back leg into the target and standing leg into the ground. The supporting leg doesn't fully straighten as that would affect the root but it does add a little bit of upward pushing power even as it stays relaxed down. This takes some practice.

You can also utilise stored power. As you stand in the dragon stance preparing to kick, pull your front (soon to be kicking) leg backwards against the ground but without moving it. Then as you raise the leg those muscles involved in pulling it backwards are already tense and doing the job. The kick will be faster although you will have less control over it once it has been released. It is like pulling back a tree branch then letting go of it to release the stored power.

Practice your back kick regularly alongside your front kick. This will not only give you an extra powerful weapon to use but also strengthen your hamstrings, gluteals (buttock muscles) and lower back, all of which tend to be weak on most people.

Chapter 16.
Effortless Throwing

Taking them down

Throws should really be an important part of any martial artist's arsenal of techniques. With a little practice throws can be applied quickly, they have the advantage of surprise and can be devastating.

Throws should be practiced until they are effortless. Throwing somebody to the ground should take no more effort than walking while swinging your arms around. For this to happen, it is vital that you have a solid, rooted stance at the point where you are applying the throw. Remember that the force that builds up between you when you apply the throw is going to take the path of least resistance therefore whoever is the least stable is the one who will be thrown. You need to be in balance and rooted downwards so that your opponent moves around you and you remain rooted to the ground until your opponent is on the floor. The throws you will learn in this book use either the horse stance or dragon stance. Train these stances first before attempting the throws otherwise you will be using too much force in your upper body to try and throw your partner down instead of relaxing the upper body and using your rooted stance.

Throws should, if necessary, incapacitate the opponent. I believe one of the main reasons why many martial artists don't include throws in their arsenal is that they are used to seeing wrestling tournaments and aikido demonstrations where somebody is thrown and then quickly rolls back onto their feet again. What's the point in learning to throw somebody if they can quickly get back up and attack you again? These aren't proper throws but demonstrations done purely for entertainment. A proper throw is one that it is impossible to roll out of, indeed it's unlikely anybody would be getting up again quickly afterwards. This can be achieved in five ways.

- The opponent is twisted or their limbs are tied up somehow during the throw so that they land badly

- The opponent is thrown and then struck once or several times before they hit the ground

- The throw is done at an increased speed so that the opponent is literally smashed into the ground

- With practice, you can judge fairly precisely where the opponent will land so you can choose to give them an uncomfortable landing in, say, a bed of nettles or on the edge of a kerb.

- While throwing you grab and keep hold of your opponent's arm so that you can control them while they are on the ground. This prevents them from rolling away or using ground fighting techniques.

None of the throws you will learn in my books or classes are ones that it would be possible to roll out of and stand back up again.

The ground fighting myth

I know this section is going to be controversial but I'll say it nevertheless. In combat you should never, ever follow your opponent to the floor. There is an often-cited theory in martial arts circles that 'most fights go to the ground'. Therefore, you need to be adept at ground fighting. It is true that most fights in the ring go to the ground because they are between two people of similar training in the same environment who aiming to score points through submission.

Real life combat, which is what this book deals with, is not like that. In real life, it is not so common for both participants to go to the ground. Certainly, one of them is likely to as they are punched, thrown or dragged to the ground but not so often do two men wrestle each other on the ground. I'm not saying it doesn't happen but it is something to be avoided at all costs. Why? Simply because a lot of real life conflict is done by guys who are showing off their prowess to their mates or a girl. Inevitably they won't be on their own as they need someone to show off to. If you go to the ground their mates, who may have been standing back before, will join in the sport of kicking you while you're down.

While you are on the floor your ability to use whole body power and leverage are severely restricted. Whole body power requires that your skeleton be upright and aligned with gravity. When you are on the ground a whole different set of skills come into play. Unless you have been trained in grappling skills and are absolutely certain that no bystanders will want to jump in then don't go to the floor.

No amount of ground fighting training can prepare you for six guys laying the boot in.

My philosophy is simple. Never, ever willingly go to the ground. I often see people doing 'sacrifice' throws. The clue is in the name people. Why sacrifice yourself just to take someone to the floor when there are far easier ways that enable you to keep your feet and maintain control? Don't do them. Don't even bother learning them. If you learn something you may be tempted to try it. They may be good for the ring but nowhere else. If your stances are good and you are rooted down most people will find it very hard indeed to take you to the ground. This is something we have tried many times in practice and the students have found it virtually impossible to take each other down as long as they maintain a well aligned root.

The other important point about not going down is to be careful when you throw anyone that you don't end up on top of them. When somebody is falling, they will instinctively grab whatever is around them to stop themselves from hitting the floor. It is likely they will grab a part of your body or clothing to try and stabilise themselves. This could easily end up dragging you down with them.

The best way to defend against this is again to ensure your ending stance is stable and that you are not leaning forward. Always maintain a straight back when throwing and never lean forward as you throw someone.

The three elements to a throw

There are three parts to any throwing move:

The entry.

These are the moves you make that get you into a position where a throw is possible. Virtually all failed attempts at throws are because the defender was in the wrong position when he attempted the throw. Generally, to get into the best position you are moving off the line of attack and towards your opponent's centre. The closer your centre is to his, the more leverage you can apply so the easier the throw becomes.

You need to get close during the entry so you are using your legs to get you into position rather than keep you stable. Your arms should be directing your opponent's arms out of the way and, if possible, grabbing them so that you can control him when he is on the floor.

The throw itself.

Any throw involves moving your opponent so that their upper body is no longer over their legs so gravity takes over and they go down. During the throw itself, you will need to drop into a stable, rooted stance so that the force you apply during the throw doesn't move you. When working with a partner just take them to the point of no return and let them fall to the floor or mat. Obviously if done for real you can accelerate the movement and slam your attacker hard onto the ground.

The follow up.

Many people now train in ground fighting so you need to be sure that your attacker isn't going to kick, grab or sweep you while they're down. Luckily this is fairly simple.

Most of the throws I teach involve maintaining a hold on one of the attacker's arms so that, as they fall, they can be quickly manipulated into a safe position. By knowing where to stand or squat in relation to their body and how to apply effective wrist and elbow locks you can quite easily prevent counter attacks from the floor.

Throws are fun to learn and can be so useful in self-defence situations. You can quickly put a person into a position on the floor where they are no longer any kind of threat to you. Alternatively, you can slam them into the ground and hurt or injure them badly. As with everything when you have learned the basics then you can adapt them to your needs.

Points to remember when throwing:

- Use leverage rather than force
- Never follow your opponent to the floor
- Use a good, upright stance
- Control them when they're down

Dragon Throw

The dragon throw is usually the first throw that students learn. This is because it's effective and easy to do. You can do lots of things wrong during this throw and it should still work. Obviously the better you do it the more effortless and powerful it becomes. As with all skills it should be practiced with a compliant partner first until you have the positioning of the feet and hands correct and can throw effortlessly. After that the partner should become progressively more resistant and offer less predictable attacks. A throw like this one will work on most people, provided you can get in close enough. That's where your yin and yang circles comes into their own.

This throw works best when you move in the direction of your opponent's forward foot. If their right leg is forward step to your left and vice versa. It can be adapted if you move towards their rear foot but it is more complicated to explain. The description below presumes the attacker is using their right arm to attack with the right leg forward.

How to do it

1. Block any movement with their arm using your left arm in a yang block and hold onto their wrist if possible.

2. Move in the direction of their forward leg. Step to the outside of their forward foot. Your foot should be alongside theirs around six inches to a foot away. Keep your forward knee well bent for stability.

3. Keep your blocking arm at least eighteen inches from your chest. Don't let it collapse in as you step forward.

4. Keeping your front leg bent and your weight on your front leg bring your back leg between your front leg and their forward leg and move it forward until it is behind their front leg.

5. At the same time put your right arm across their body onto their left shoulder. Not you are in position for the throw.

6. In one move sweep your right foot directly back taking their forward leg out from under them.

7. At the same time turn your hips to the left and sweep your right arm forward and down so that your fingertips point to the ground in front of you. Your opponent will drop to the ground with their head in front of your left foot. If you have managed to keep hold of their wrist with your left hand you are now in a position to apply a wrist lock to prevent them trying ground fighting techniques.

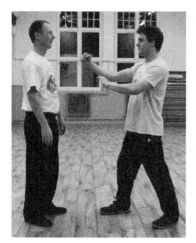

Attacker throws punch

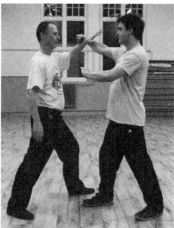

Step to left and block punch

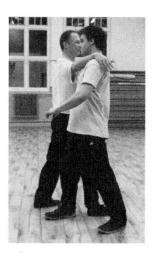

Step right leg behind
and put arm on shoulder

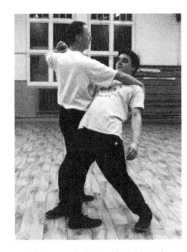
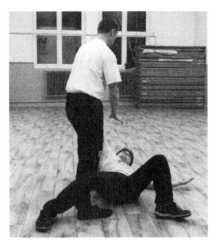

Sweep right leg back and right arm forward and down

Keep hold of attacker's wrist with left hand

Notice that, as with all our throws, there is no way for the opponent to roll out of it or get back up easily. Being able to maintain control of someone once you've thrown them to the floor may be an essential skill in certain circumstances.

Although you can, and should, practice the movement on its own it is clearly best if you can find a partner to practice on. With throw techniques, most people will react in the same way ie go straight to the floor so what will happen next is predictable. This isn't so with joint locks or pressure points etc. Joint locks are dependent on the opponent's habitual way of moving and patterns of tension in their body. Throws simply take their base away from under their upper body and let gravity do the rest. It only takes a few goes to get this to work well. So, grab a friend and try it. Don't expect it to work for you if you've never practised it.

Forward Horse Throw

The forward horse throw is similar to the dragon throw above except that you end up in a horse stance instead of a dragon stance.

How to do it

1. Start with a yang block with the left arm then step to the outside of their front foot.

2. Step forward with your back foot and bring it behind their body into a horse stance.

3. Place your right arm onto their left shoulder.

4. Throw them by lowering your horse stance and moving your right arm diagonally forward and down until the fingers are pointing at ground between your feet and just in front of you.

145

As with the dragon stance try to keep hold of their right arm with your left hand to give you control of them when they land.

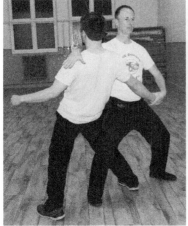 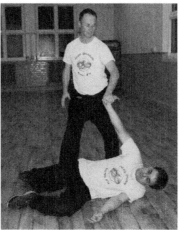

Throwing position for horse throw. Lower stance and direct right arm down and forward to throw

Final position for throw keeping control of opponent through wrist lock

The most common mistakes beginners make with this throw are firstly, they let their right knee collapse inward as the opponent falls. Keep your knees apart as you throw, don't allow the structure of your horse stance to collapse. Secondly, they commonly lean forward as they throw in an effort to use the weight of the upper body to assist the throw. This is not only unnecessary but will leave you in a position where you are off balance and can be easily pulled to the floor on top of the person you have just thrown.

Backward Horse Throw

The backward horse throw is slightly more complicated than the other two. However, it is the throw we have been able to perform most successfully while sparring. As I mentioned previously it is almost impossible to get a set technique to work during the constantly changing circumstances of sparring. This throw could be the exception to that rule as it can be applied quickly and without warning. You simply lead their hand across their body, step behind and drop them. They're often on the floor before they realise what happened. Although that is assuming you are sparring with bridged hands rather than in the less effective boxers guard. I shall explain more in Part Three.

As with the forward horse throw you perform the move from the horse stance except this time you throw them backward over your horse stance rather than forward.

How to do it

Again, we will assume they are forward on their right leg. There are two ways of doing this move depending on your height relative to your opponent's height.

If you're around the same height or taller than your opponent:

1. Move their right arm inward with a yang block with your right arm or a yin block with your left arm. Either way you are moving to the outside of their leading arm.

2. Step your left leg behind their forward right leg and drop into a good horse stance.

3. Put your left arm over their right shoulder and across their chest with your palm facing away from them.

4. Sink into your stance and lead your left forearm backwards and downwards slightly and they will be pushed backwards over your horse stance.

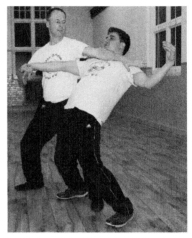

Throwing position for attacker who is same size or smaller than you.

This should be practiced until it is familiar and smooth and then you can speed up the process of getting into the right position.

If your opponent is somewhat taller than you so that you can't put your left arm over their shoulder:

1. Block their arm and step behind in the same way but keep a hold of their wrist with your right hand.

2. Put your left arm under their shoulder and across their chest or belly instead of over. There is a risk here that they might back elbow you in the face so lift their right arm over your head and behind your neck. At this point you can safely let go of their arm.

3. Sink into your stance and lead your left arm back and down. They will be on the floor before they can even think of grabbing your neck.

Another alternative is to use your left hand to lead their right arm across their body while you step behind with your left leg and throw them while still keeping their right arm across their body. This is an excellent alternative as it is often faster to get into and prevents them using their right arm to break their fall.

The only real disadvantage to this throw is that, unlike the previous two throws it doesn't enable you to keep hold of their arm so that you can control them when they're down. They will fall to your left and slightly behind you. It is also not as powerful as the previous two throws as you cannot slam them into the ground with the power of your chest and waist muscles. Other than that, it's a useful throw to learn.

Chapter 17.
Connected Power in Kung Fu

In this, the final chapter of this section I will show you the basics of how to develop the connected power that enables you to create huge force without effort and by barely moving at all. This is the 'secret' that so many martial artists over the centuries have sought but often haven't found.

The good news is that the 'secret' is here for you today. The bad news is that this knowledge is utterly useless to you unless you practice it. By that I mean practice it every single day for years and years to come. You see other martial artists either didn't know the simple principles I'll show you here or they did know but didn't want to spend years developing it so they looked for shortcuts.

I can tell you here and now that there aren't any shortcuts to developing effortless power.

Don't believe, and certainly don't pay for anyone or any system that claims you can develop great power in a matter of weeks or so. As the great Professor Cheng Man Ching once said, each training session is like putting a single piece of paper on top of a stack of papers. Each one may seem to make no difference but gradually, over time, the stack gets higher and higher. As will your skill level.

The two power movements

There are only two movements a human being can do that produce any real power. They are simple movements but require endless practice. When we need to produce a powerful movement, for example if you want to strike or move another person then the technique should include one or preferably both of these movements. You should learn to use these movements more and more in everyday life and to use them all the time in your kung fu practice to ensure that sufficient power is generated to make the techniques work. It is often said that it is better to learn half a dozen techniques well and with power than to learn a thousand techniques poorly.

The two power movements involve the biggest muscles of the body. These are situated in the lower part of the body and in the centre. Typically, most people prefer to use the muscles of the upper body - the shoulders, arms, chest and upper back. These are relatively small and weak muscles so require a lot of training to make them strong.

It is better, and quicker, to learn to use the bigger muscles of the lower body first when moving instead of the smaller muscles near the top. You can virtually double your power instantly by moving properly. What takes the time and practice is the precise and subtle coordination of different parts of the body to create fluid and connected power.

Transfer the weight

As I said earlier these two movements are seemingly very simple. The first movement is to transfer your body weight from one leg to the other. This involves using the muscles of one leg to push your body across to be supported by the muscles of the other leg. You start with your supporting leg bent at the knee and the unweighted leg straight, or almost straight. Then you gradually straighten the supporting leg and bend the unweighted leg and transfer the weight across. It is important that you keep your weight as low as you can throughout the movement. Don't allow your stance to raise up as you cross then drop again on the other side, keep it the same height throughout.

This movement can be done either with the feet side by side, somewhat more than shoulder width apart. This drives the body across and is useful for sideways punches. Alternatively, and more usefully it should also be done with one leg in front of the other. The most beneficial way being from a forward dragon stance back into a tiger stance then forward into dragon again.

Keep your upper body upright throughout the movement with your head over your hips. Don't be tempted to lean side to side or backwards and forwards in even the smallest degree. Also keep your hips in a neutral position throughout with your sacrum relaxed down to ensure the upper body is strongly connected to the powerful movement of the legs.

The art of t'ai chi chuan involves a lot of movement from one bent leg to the other. Over time the legs can support more weight and the stance can be gradually lowered. It is largely this movement from one weighted (yin) leg to the unweighted (yang) leg that gives the art both its name and its power.

Turn the waist

The second movement also seems quite simple. The movement is as described, simply twist your body from the waist from one side to the other. Gradually the hips open up allowing a greater range of movement and the legs become more involved allowing for more power.

When you twist your body to the side it is like a coiled spring. There is a build-up of potential energy waiting to be unleashed into your next technique. As I mentioned in the section on general conditioning you should differentiate between turning the waist and turning the hips. Turning the waist is a smaller movement than turning the hips but a lot more powerful. That small, yet powerful movement is a key aspect of generating effortless power and in being able to throw around larger and stronger opponents than yourself with simple movements that are small, yet effortless.

Move from the centre

To accomplish the above two key movements successfully it is essential that you learn to move from your centre. Remember that your body has a lot of joints in it. Whenever you try to move from anywhere other than your centre that part of the body will lead the movement. When that happens, you will no longer be aligned with gravity and the movement won't be coordinated throughout your body.

Typically, it is the upper body that leads. Most people walk with their head thrust forward or down so the upper body is bent slightly forward. They look down at the ground, oblivious to what is going on around them. With every step they take they are accumulating tension all down the back of their body from their neck down to their feet. This tension must be there to stop them from falling forward under their own weight. Once you learn to move from the centre you will walk more upright, look more poised and more confident, be more aware of your environment, look less like a victim and be less tense when you arrive.

Most fighters lean forward when they punch. It is a natural reaction as the arm connects to the torso near the top so they follow their arm forward as they punch. The idea is that they get the weight of the body behind the punch. But, if they are leaning forward they can only get part of their body weight behind it. By standing up straight, using your legs, rooting into the ground, and moving from the centre far more force is available.

So, when you are focusing on the key movements of transferring your weight and turning your waist focus on doing so from your centre and not from your upper body.

Practice one movement

It is better to learn one or two movements well than a thousand movements poorly.

To learn to generate power effectively means coordinating your entire body together in many subtle ways. The only way to do this is to focus on one key movement and do it over and over again tens of thousands of times and to focus on coordinating and relaxing different aspects of it.

To a certain extent, it doesn't matter what movement you choose but it should preferably be one that involves a transfer of weight from one leg to the other, a turn of the waist in both directions and a circular movement of the arms. Your arms need to be carried by the movement of the legs and waist. Appropriate movements would include 'grasping the sparrow's tail' from t'ai chi chuan or 'single palm change' from bagua-zhang or any full body movement from whatever style you practice. My personal fa-vourite is moving the body backward and forward from a tiger to forward dragon (with-out moving the back foot) while turning the waist and doing yin circles with the arms. This is almost identical to 'brush knee twist step' in t'ai chi chuan. I do many repeti-tions on one side then repeat on the other side. When you do it correctly staying relaxed and moving from the centre it brings in a lot of chi energy so you should feel your hands tingling and eventually your whole body will fill with energy.

When practicing this one movement focus on the following:

- Coordinate your arms together then your arms and legs together.

- Keep your whole body as relaxed and rooted down throughout the whole movement as possible.

- Breathe easily and naturally deep into your abdomen.

- Maintain a smoothness of movement.

- Ensure that when one part of your body is fully forward that all parts are and that you aren't leaning forward even slightly. The same for when you are fully on the back leg. Don't lean back and smoothly make the change of direction involving your whole body.

- Maintain an awareness of what is going on inside your body. Try to feel where your weight is, where each part of the body is in relation to the other parts and see if you can feel any movement of energy.

PART 3 – TACTICS

Chapter 18.
Gaining Control

In Part three we will look at how and when to use the skills you learned in the previous section. We will look at the psychology of violence and self-defence. We will look at some useful tactics for real life situations. We will also look at how to use your newfound skills to improve your health and make your life easier.

Real combat is nothing like most martial arts training.

Don't expect your martial arts training to be the same as real life violence. In martial arts classes, you know who each other is and you've become friends over the months and years. So, a common class scenario is where your class mate offers you his arm and you grab it carefully and throw him to the ground then enquire if he's ok afterwards. Real combat isn't like this. It's brutal, it's fast and it's unfair. Don't expect people to behave in any way like your friends or classmates would. In combat, they want to hurt you for real so you must be mentally prepared for this. Classes are good in that they get you over the shock of physical, hard contact with another person but they can't simulate real life violence.

One critical point to remember is that, in all human conflict, the person who most believes they will win usually does

Oh my God, you are being threatened with actual physical violence. What should you do? Most people have never faced real physical aggression before or if they have they found it traumatising to say the least. Good self-defence should give you the skills not only to deal with the attack but also how you deal with the aftermath. Being attacked is extremely traumatising. Not just to your physical self but it also damages your confidence and destroys your ego. If you allow it to affect you then it can get stuck in your mind and in your physiology for many years afterwards, even your whole life and affect every decision you make. So, the first and most important lesson you need to learn is how to deal with the emotional aspects of violence or the threat of violence.

The rising tide of panic

The Chinese say that when we panic the energy in our body rises. It comes up out of your feet and legs and your knees start to shake. It rises up above your waist and abdominal breathing becomes impossible. Your breathing gets higher and faster as your energy and panic rise. Your chest feels like it's being squeezed in a vice, your breath gets so high it feels like you're choking and cannot breathe anymore. This is a classic panic attack. The energy rises into your head and prevents you from thinking clearly. It also causes tunnel vision which prevents you from using your peripheral vision to see threats coming at you from the sides. So, you cannot see clearly, you cannot think clearly, you can barely breathe, your body is fighting itself from within and is locked tight with tension. You cannot put a coherent thought or movement together. You are now the perfect victim and are utterly helpless to any incoming attack.

You need to counter this rising panic or, better still, stop it before it starts. Good kung fu training isn't just to make you physically strong but also helps to keep you emotionally stable. Just follow the principles that have been discussed in this book and you will be in a far better state to deal with the potential violent situation in front of you.

The first thing to do is bend your knees slightly and feel the ground beneath your feet. This will prevent the loss of feeling in your legs and enable you to move quickly when needed. Now you need to consciously relax downwards. Imagine a wave of relaxation from the top of your head going down through your body. Feel your shoulders drop, relax your sacrum down, drop your elbows etc. You should practice this regularly when you are in a relaxed state. If you can't do this when you're relaxed then you have no chance of doing it when you're highly stressed and under threat of attack. Consciously breathe into your lower abdomen. This will help you to relax and bring in the air and resources you need to move effectively. These measures alone should prevent the energy from rising, give you control of your legs and enable you to plan and move as necessary.

Now that you have manipulated your physiology to prevent panic building up within you, focus on expanding yourself outwards. Imagine yourself getting bigger and bigger and your opponent shrinking before you. This will add immeasurably to your courage and the act of expanding outward will prevent fear from causing you to contract inward. I will talk more about this concept of expanding in future books although it was already covered quite comprehensively in "Stress Proof Your Body".

Being able to relax under pressure is the single most important thing you can learn. Stress and tension are killers. They destroy lives and make you miserable. But it doesn't have to be that way. Kung fu teaches a range of principles and skills to make such tension a thing of the past. Read my book 'Stress Proof Your Body' for much more information on how to use these and other principles to deal with pressure and help you live a longer, happier, and less stressful life.

The three types of attacker

Attackers tend to come in three types that I call the judge, the predator and the show-off.

- The judge is the guy who thinks you have wronged him somehow. You spilled his drink, you cut him up on the road, whatever it may be. You have broken one of the rules in his personal rulebook and he has set himself up as judge, jury, and executioner. The easiest thing to do is be the bigger man, or woman and apologise. Not just apologise but explain why you did it in a simple sentence. "Sorry pal, you were in my blind spot and I didn't see you there. Hope you're ok?" That kind of thing is often enough to avert violence but not always. Some people are plain sociopaths and can't be reasoned with.

- Predators want something that you have, your money, your phone, your body and so on. They are looking for victim types – people with their head down, not looking where they're going and with their mind somewhere else entirely. When they have found such a person they get in close without you being aware of it then attack in a method designed to overwhelm you. Alternatively, they threaten with or use a weapon such as a knife that will overwhelm you mentally and demand your possessions. The way to avoid them is to stay aware and don't let anyone too close if you can help it. If you feel that someone is possibly going to mug or rape you then try to stay calm and look them in the face and imprint their image on your mind. The last thing a predator wants is for someone to recognise them in a line-up later or anyone who looks like they might put up a fight. Often the mere act of being aware and staring at them is enough for them to realise that you're not worth mugging.

- The show-off is the third dangerous character. He wants to show how tough he is to his mates or to a girl. To do this he will come on strong and try to antagonise you. Show-offs tend to pick on larger guys as there's not many kudos on picking on a smaller person than himself. If such a guy is trying to intimidate you it will likely trigger one of the two primary emotions of anger or fear. Anger will drive you forward to recklessly attack the attacker. Fear will pull you back or freeze you and drain you of the resources you need to survive the encounter. Neither emotion is helpful so you must curb these emotions and show nothing to the show-off. Stay balanced and upright and relax downwards into your feet. Anger will make you lean forward whereas fear will make you lean backwards. Keeping yourself upright helps you to prevent the trigger of these dangerous emotions.

The three types of martial arts

We covered the three most likely types of attacker but it's also worth looking at the three main types of martial artist as well. This will help you should you be attacked by someone with some fight training. By understanding the strengths and weaknesses of the three types of combat training you will be better able to know what is likely to work and what isn't against these different fighting camps.

There are hundreds of martial arts in the world and each of them uses specific tactics to cope with the rigours of combat. All martial arts focus on different things, no single martial style can hope to be able to deal with every type of situation, every type of attack, every weapon, every set of circumstances and so on.

In particular, each of them has to come to terms with the stability-mobility continuum. This means that the more stable you are the less mobile you are and vice versa. Both are needed in combat - stability to give efficient power to your movements and mobility to get you out of danger and move you into the right position to counterattack quickly.

There have been many attempts to categorise martial arts but I think the most useful is to divide them into three camps – the kick-punch camp, the grappling camp and the stance based camp.

- The kick-punch camp favours mobility over stability. They stay light on their feet and dance around in front of the opponent weaving out of the way of attacks and looking for gaps in the defence which they then spring forward to exploit. Fighters in this camp are always strikers and kickers. They don't use throws or joint locks as these require a solid contact with the ground to provide the necessary leverage. This lack of contact with the ground means they are unable to develop whole body power so they need to develop local power. Local power comes from the muscles local to the movement. E.g. their strikes come mostly from the arm and shoulder muscles and less from the back, waist and legs. Examples from this camp include boxing, kickboxing, taekwondo and muay thai among others.

- The grappling camp specialises in keeping the centre of gravity low and taking their opponent to the ground. Once there they aim to immobilise the opponent or cause significant pain and joint damage. Grapplers low stance and willingness to take the fight to the ground can make them difficult to defend against. However, it also makes them vulnerable to multiple attackers as, in grappling, all focus is on one man and grappling with more than one at a time is almost impossible. The grappling camp includes judo, jujitsu, BJJ and all kinds of wrestling.

- The stance based camp aims for a balance of mobility and stability. The stance camp uses upright stances where the body is relaxed down onto the ground. This gives added power to all movements as the whole body works together - arms, legs, waist, back etc. and is firmly rooted to the ground for maximum efficiency of movement. At the moment when force is being applied the whole body becomes as stable as possible so that the forces move the opponent not the one in the good stance. With practice, the root can be lifted for maximum mobility or dropped for maximum power extremely quickly to give the relaxed power and freedom of movement that is often necessary in combat. The stance camp differs from the kick-punch camp in that at least one foot is almost always on the ground and the entire body weight is balanced and aligned through that foot. It is very rare for both feet to be off the ground as is common with in many combat sports. It also differs from the grappling camp in that the body posture is upright instead of leaning forward which limits what the practitioner can see and how he can move. A martial artist who uses stances well can use them in any kind of combat - throws, locks, kicks, strikes and so on. This added versatility makes them a formidable fighter.

I have only ever trained in the stance camp but it seems to me to be the one that is most effective for real combat. The kick-punch camp's lack of whole body power and the grappler's lack of defence against multiple opponents are inherent weaknesses that cannot be overcome through additional training. Many boxers and kick boxers etc. may argue that they do use their whole body. But they don't in the same way that stance based martial artists do. Boxers and others from that camp tend to lean forward behind their punch. In doing so they are putting themselves off balance at the point of impact so they aren't using their full body weight behind the punch, only a part of it.

This is why I teach a stance based martial art. I refuse to teach anything that I can see an inherent weakness in and I see these weaknesses scattered throughout many of the martial arts I've seen. Most of my long-term students have previous martial arts training and they are full of stories about techniques they've been taught that nobody can get to work effectively including the teachers. I have personally tested every skill I teach. They work for real, against resisting opponents. All they take is some practice and an understanding of the principles involved.

I believe stance based martial skills are the most difficult to defend against but probably also the least likely to attack. The correct postural alignment training that is required for stance based martial arts requires you to be relaxed in mind and body, and someone who is relaxed and balanced is unlikely to go around starting fights. Fights are started by people who have something to prove or there's something they want that they will risk getting hurt for. More often than not, it all starts with a push.

Don't push back

The most common prelude to any fight is being pushed or grabbed. What happens when somebody pushes you? You either give in to their push or you push back. It's instinctive, you don't think about it you just do it. It's an automatic reaction. But it's a reaction that doesn't serve you well. If you push back at every pressure then life becomes a constant struggle and the greater force will always win. Pushing back also drains you of power and energy as a lot is wasted in trying to maintain that resisting force. In kung fu we learn to use our power more intelligently. We learn that there are alternatives to pushing back, each of which is preferable.

Offer no resistance yet stay balanced. This will likely unbalance your opponent and make a fast counter-attack more likely to work. T'ai chi chuan has an entire discipline, push hands, that specialises in getting you to overcome the natural tendency to push back and instead to offer no resistance to an attack, to remain soft, yet in constant contact with the attacker.

Once you are in relaxed contact with your attacker you can redirect his incoming force. The circular movements that we teach enable you to merge with the incoming force and circle it harmlessly away from you or even back into the assailant. By using a circular motion, you can maintain contact with his attacking limb for longer and so have a better chance of grabbing and manipulating that limb. Remember that, although they may be striking with all their force, that force is targeted in only one direction and towards one point in space - their target. It is easy and takes almost no effort to redirect that force as has been proved many times by redirecting an attacking arm with just one finger.

Alternatively, stand in a stable yet relaxed posture and allow the force to go through you and into the ground. This is called rooting and enables the kung fu practitioner to absorb force from different directions yet remain relaxed, balanced, and able to counter-attack instantly in any direction. It is important that no attempt is made to physically resist the force as that will lock up your muscles and prevent fast and easy escape or counterattack movements. To learn how to do this see the earlier section on stance training. When doing this you form your strong structure first before you make physical contact with your opponent. This can be done instantaneously with a little practice. If you try to form a good structure while he is putting pressure on you it will be much harder and could be too late to defend against a strong attack. It is best to create the structure before the attack and if possible move to the side of your opponent while maintaining that strong, expanded posture. Now you are in an excellent position to counter-attack.

Each of these alternative countermeasures to an incoming force needs to be practised as the instinctive need to push back is strongly ingrained in all of us. Regular practice with a partner at these physical disciplines gives you the ability to cope with other pressures using the same tactics. Next time someone is giving you a hard time verbally - you're involved in an argument that you didn't want or being pressured to do something you don't want to do then remember these tactics.

Don't resist, stay balanced and redirect

Learn to offer no resistance yet stay emotionally balanced inside and physically balanced so that your head stays over your feet. When you are under pressure you resist emotionally first and this turns into physical resistance which locks up your muscles. Stay emotionally and physically balanced and you will be in a better position to see the new situation for what it is and find ways to deal with it.

Most confrontations and stressful events trigger one of two opposing emotions in us - fear or anger. Anger causes tightening in the front of the body so we instinctively lean forward ready to lash out at the cause of our anger. Fear causes tension in the back of the body so we are prepared to move backwards quickly. It causes us to lean backwards. Neither of these are good as both of them take us out of balance and into a vulnerable position. Learn to stand balanced and stay balanced and you will be less likely to feel fear or anger in stressful situations. This may take off some of the pressure and allow a compromise situation to be reached. This also helps you to see the situation from the other person's point of view (empathy) and so may help you to resolve the situation without conflict.

Another option for dealing with pressure in combat or in life is to redirect the pressure away from you. You should always start off by moving in the same direction as the pressure before you redirect it. If you are having an argument with someone you should start by agreeing with them first. This will soften their stance and enable you to gently redirect them towards your own point of view. By agreeing with the person who's giving you a hard time you avoid the clash of people pushing in opposite directions and who stop listening to each other and waste their efforts solely on proving that they are right and the other is wrong.

We've all been there. Nobody emerges better off from such confrontations. Redirecting the pressure means merging with their point of view then gradually changing the outcome into one that is favourable to both of you. If you have tried offering no resistance, if you have tried redirecting the force away from you and still the pressure is on then put yourself in a physically balanced position and mentally relax every part of your body downwards. This will enable you to anchor yourself during the storm so that you can survive it emotionally intact. In this way, you can prevent yourself from being caught up in the other person's emotional drama and so end up doing or saying things that you may later regret. Again, this is a fabulously useful skill that everyone should learn and enables you to maintain your personal power when someone else is trying to rob you of it.

During conflict, particularly where violence may be involved many people worry that their voice will give away their anxiety. This is a real possibility. A voice that's weak and an octave higher than normal doesn't sound cool or authoritative. It is usually best to say nothing unless you are sure that your voice will be firm, calm and assured. Your voice will give away any internal fear or tension you will probably be feeling so if you don't trust your voice, don't use it and say nothing.

Just remember, whenever you feel threatened in any way you should take a relaxed stance and show an attitude that is neutral i.e. neither passive nor aggressive as both overt passivity or aggression could trigger an attack. Keep your hands in a position where they can be used but aren't overly aggressive. Don't have them behind your back or in your pockets but equally, don't adopt any kind of fighting pose. The best thing to do is extend them out in front of you with palms out in a pacifying nature. This doesn't look aggressive but it places your hands between your attacker and you and means you don't have to move far to block any incoming attacks.

Connect and Control

When faced with an incoming attack your first priority should be to control the space between yourself and your opponent. Your next priority should be to control the opponent himself by connecting your arms to his. This is called bridging and is an essential element to training in many martial arts.

In many combat sports and in most sparring, there is a tendency to engage briefly with the opponent and then disengage again. Then to continue the pattern of engaging and disengaging. This is dangerous and draws out the fight needlessly. While you are disengaged you are allowing your opponent to regain his strength and focus. You cannot predict what he will do next and cannot control him. When you are engaged you can feel what he is doing better than you can see and, to a large degree, you can control his movements. Bridging quickly teaches you that the best strategy is to engage and then stay engaged until the fight is won (or lost).

While you are maintaining contact you shouldn't need to look at your opponent but should be able to use the feedback from the touch of his hands to know exactly what the opponent is doing. Learning to feel the changes in your opponent and respond to your sense of touch i.e. fighting without looking is a great skill to develop. You will find that your sense of touch is faster and more accurate than your eyes. It doesn't take much practice for a person to be able to strike faster than you can see. But, if you're in contact with the strike as it comes in then you can feel and react to it much faster than you could if you were relying on your eyes alone to see the incoming punch. There are three other reasons why learning to fight without looking can be important.

- Many people use facial expressions, staring eyes and the tone of their voice to intimidate, to instil fear or anger in their victims. By not looking directly at your assailant you are less likely to be hypnotised or psyched out like a mouse with a cobra.

- Rarely does a person start a fight on his own these days. Often, he will be part of a group. Being able to make contact then control your assailant without looking at him means you are free to look around you, assess the situation and environment, see who are his allies and who are your own, find the exits, find objects that could help you or help your assailant etc.

- Finally, not looking at your assailant signifies that he is beneath your contempt and not worth bothering with. This is psychologically damaging to them and likely to arouse their own fear and anger - exactly what they were trying to do to you.

Sticky hands

To practice this skill, you need a partner. The basic exercise is simple - you just touch your arms together and follow each other's movements using as little force as possible. If your opponent raises his arm you stay attached and raise yours. If he pushes his arm towards you don't resist it but move yours back at the same speed and maintaining the same pressure. To start with you will feel pressure building up between your arms as you habitually resist each other. When this happens, and it will, you may need to break contact and start again with a lighter touch. You absolutely need to prevent this tension building up. Your objective is to be able to follow them without any effort or resistance and be able to lightly redirect their incoming movements. If there is tension in your arms when you do this it minimises how well you can sense their movements with your arm or hand. It also prevents you from moving freely to adapt and redirect their movements. This will slow down your reaction speed. The tenser you are the jerkier your responses will be. The excess tension also continually drains you of energy and power and you need to conserve your power in life as in combat. Finally tension in your arms and shoulders will make you top heavy and prevent you using your whole body effectively to deliver real power when you need it. Remember, if your arms feel strong and powerful then you are doing it wrong. The power should come from your waist and legs. There should be no feeling of power in the arms at all. If there is they cannot respond quickly to your opponent's actions.

To master sticky hands takes years of practice

Sticky hands takes a long time to become proficient at but even after just one session you will have significantly increased your ability to respond quickly to the sensation of your opponent moving towards you. Sticky hands practice keeps your mind in your body and focused constantly on what you and your partner are doing. You cannot daydream in this practice so it keeps you rooted mentally to the here and now. As I mentioned above, when you become proficient at this practice you can control an opponent without even looking at him by staying relaxed and keeping your hands lightly on his arms to redirect his attacks. He will find this enormously frustrating as it is difficult for even an experienced martial artist to put together a useful attack when the opponent sticks to every move he makes. Many Chinese martial arts have their own versions of this exercise – t'ai chi has push hands, wing chun has chi sao, bagua has rou shou and so on.

Working with a partner

 As you will have gathered by now having at least one training partner is essential to learning kung fu. Ideally you should have more than one as everybody is different and will react differently to everything you do to them. If you just have the one you may be lulled into thinking that, as your moves work on your partner, they will work on everyone. This is dangerous thinking. They won't and you don't want to find that out the hard way in real street violence.

Most of your training, at least 70% of it should be done on your own. Only when you have practiced a move until it is very familiar and has been hardwired into your body should you try it with a partner. The reason for this is that, when working with a partner people tend to focus on the end rather than the means. For example, they want their partner to go down when they throw them so they focus on the partner and try to push them down with their upper body. They forget all the principles of correct body usage and just focus on throwing them down as best they can. Their body isn't aligned properly, they aren't using their stance to make the move work etc. So, they end up having to use a lot of force to take them down when it could and should be effortless.

Solo practice should be 70% of your training time.
Partner practice should be the other 30%.

Practice the movement on your own many, many times first and then, when you have your partner there stay focused on yourself. You can almost forget the partner is there and just be aware of moving your body from the centre and using your legs. Your partner will go down easily and you will be amazed at how little effort you had to put into it.

When working with a partner focus on the process not the result.

Your partner should be compliant to start with and offer a simple arm or leg for you to work with to get the positioning right for the technique. Once you have the positioning right and can perform the movement with some power and minimal effort only then should your partner become gradually more resistant and unpredictable in their attack. A partner who attacks fast and hard before you have learned the technique against an unresisting attack isn't going to teach you anything. Make the attacks and your responses slow and smooth and gradually speed up. There is no rush. As you and your partner become more advanced there will be attacks they throw at you that don't allow you to do the technique you want to practice. Maybe they are moving too fast or their body is in the wrong position, or yours is. It's best you find this out in the practice room than for real on the street. This is where you need to learn to either adapt your moves to suit the circumstances or abandon the technique completely and try something else. Obviously, this decision needs to be made instantaneously.

Be smooth

When using a partner as with solo training always move slowly to start. A lot of what learning kung fu is about is letting go of bad movement habits and learning to move in more efficient ways. When new students start at my school and begin practicing with a partner much of what they learned during solo practice, the principles of alignment and moving the whole body as one unit go out of the window. One of the most common mistakes is to try to start off their movement with a strong, fast action. This creates a jerky movement with all the force at the beginning and only momentum to carry the movement through to its completion. This is bad practice for several reasons:

- A jerky movement has all the power at the beginning of the movement and no power after that. However, often it isn't the beginning of your movement where you will meet resistance, it is part way through the movement. If all your power is at the beginning you will have some speed but no real power when you meet the real resistance.

Smooth movements maintain their power throughout the movement. Jerky movements do not.

- A jerky movement inevitably means that some parts of the body will be moving faster than others. Usually the hand movements rush ahead of the rest of the body or the hip kicks out first so you end up using just the muscles in the arms, chest and shoulders to create the force instead of using the bigger muscles lower down.

- A jerky movement automatically triggers resistance in the opponent and, because the jerky movement has no power after the initial jerk, it isn't strong enough for long enough to overcome that resistance.

Most fighters use jerky movements and aren't used to defending themselves against smooth moves.

Students usually use jerky movements in the, often erroneous belief that they need to move fast in combat. In fact, this is far from always the case. Always remember the following.

Take control, then slow down

When you are in contact with and in control of your opponent then moving at speed is neither necessary nor desirable. The thing to do is to gain control and then slow down. Once you have one or both hands on your opponent's arms or body then you have some measure of control over his movements. At this point it is connected power that will make the difference, not speed. He will be desperately trying to keep his balance while trying to figure out a defence or counter-attack while you can move him around at will. If your movements are circular he won't be able to adapt to them quick enough to put up much of a defence. This is something we have spent hundreds of hours proving in class time.

Most smooth, circular movements mean you can constantly change the speed and direction of your movement skills. You could be pulling someone forward then smoothly change to pulling them to the side then pushing them backward. They cannot easily adapt to these smooth and powerful changes of direction and invariably go to the ground.

Using your connected power means using your upper and lower body together as one unit rooted into the ground so that any movement you do uses all your body weight and the force will move whichever of you is the least stable. To do this you need to stand strong and move from your waist and legs letting your arms be carried by your centre and lower body. In this way, your movement becomes more powerful than your opponent can resist. Speed is unnecessary and will only disconnect your arms from the power that is coming up from your legs and waist. If you want to move your opponent quickly then start off slow and then accelerate the move. This gives you far more control over the speed and direction of a movement than if you were to start it fast and try to maintain the speed.

Furthermore, a movement that starts off gradually then speeds up tends not to trigger much resistance in the opponent. By the time they realise they are being moved they are already misaligned, on the move and easy to take down.

Most importantly, a smoother movement gives you complete control over the movement. You can control its speed, you can change the angle of movement during the movement and you can adapt constantly to the way your opponent is reacting to it. A jerky movement allows for none of this. Once the movement is launched the speed cannot easily be controlled nor can it change direction without significantly slowing it down first. It has virtually no power beyond the first few inches and cannot adapt to how the opponent may react to it. Techniques succeed or fail largely due to their ability to adapt to the demands placed on them.

Start slow, stay smooth then speed up.

When you have some contact with your opponent slow down and use your legs and waist to control your arms. This will give you the power to maintain control of yourself and your opponent by adapting all the time to how they move.

Now you have some general principles for how to deal physically and emotionally with a possible attack let's look at some specific techniques.

The common types of assault

According to a study compiled by police forces across Britain, the ten most common types of attack in order are:

1. Attacker pushes, defender pushes back, attacker throws a swinging punch to the head
2. A swinging punch to the head
3. Front clothing grab, one handed, followed by punch to head
4. Two handed front clothing grab, followed by headbutt
5. Two handed front clothing grab followed by knee to groin
6. Bottle, glass or ashtray swung to the head
7. A lashing kick to groin/lower legs
8. A bottle or glass jabbed to face
9. A slash with a knife, usually 3-4-inch lock-blade or kitchen knife
10. A grappling style headlock

The number 1 scenario above is one I'm sure you've seen before. The aggressor pushes or grabs his intended victim to show his dominance. This is an attempt to trigger either fear or anger in you. The attacker knows that either emotion will help him and not you. It is also an attempt to get you to throw the first punch. Then he can claim that you started it and he was just defending himself.

Do not allow anyone to put their hands on you without your permission. That is an assault. Don't allow yourself to be grabbed as when a person grabs you they have some control over you and this can make you very vulnerable. The scenarios numbered 4 and 5 above can happen instantly after you've been grabbed. If you don't block their hands away straightaway you could be in a bad way very quickly.

Three of the most common types of assault according to the list above involve a punch swung to the head. Your best defence is to develop your shield and your yang block. This involves that instantaneous creation of a strong structure I spoke about earlier and will be covered in more detail in the next book in this series. This will also protect against number 6, the bottle swung to the head.

Number 4 is a grab followed quickly by a headbutt. This can happen very quickly and is one of the reasons why you shouldn't allow anyone to grab you. A simple defence against this is to place the palm of your hand under their upper arm and push upwards and inwards. This usually dislodges their arm and bends their body backwards so that the headbutt can no longer reach. This should also protect you against number 5, the knee to the groin. An even easier alternative would be a yin block with the blade of your forearm to the outside of their grabbing arm. This will release the grip and prevent them from any fast follow up. It is easy to step forward into a throwing position from there or continue the yin circle for a striking opportunity. Read the upcoming Defences Against Grabs section for more options.

Number 7 – a kick to the lower legs is not debilitating if you are standing correctly unless it is a very hard kick (which is unlikely) or is correctly aimed at certain vulnerable points in the lower body. When your body is aligned and rooted downwards the forces acting on it are also directed downwards into the ground. This means you can train yourself to be able to withstand many strikes and kicks. Kicks to the legs are easily rooted as they are already close to the ground and your leg muscles, while holding the stance, help protect the vulnerable joints. Ignore the kicks if you can and stay relaxed or move aside from them and counter from a different direction.

A bottle or glass jabbed to the face (number 8) is the same as a direct forward strike. Your shield should protect you. Either your yin or yang circles can block this and a continuation of the circle will give you the counter attack.

Number 9 is a slash with a knife. This is clearly extremely serious and unless you are very experienced and confident you know what you're doing I wouldn't recommend engaging with this. Get out of there fast.

Number 10 is a headlock. Again, this can be debilitating but there are certain techniques that can help you escape and counter attack. These will be covered later.

Learning some simple street fighting skills can help you survive some nasty street encounters. More importantly learn not to present yourself as a victim. Don't walk around with your head down. Walk by leading from the centre rather than your head. This will keep you alert to what is going on around you and will put less stress on your body as you walk. You will look and feel more alert and confident and far less like a victim.

Chapter 19.
Defences Against Grabs

As you read earlier the most common type of attack starts with a grab or push. Usually the assailant is trying to intimidate you or possibly to get a hold so that they can follow quickly with a headbutt, swinging punch or knee to the groin. It's important that you act quickly and decisively. Fortunately, there are dozens of ways to defend against someone grabbing or pushing you. Here are a few of my favourites.

Never forget that an opponent who is intimidating you is hoping to trigger one of two reactions: anger or fear. Either of these reactions makes you less effective at defending yourself so control your emotional reactions, stay calm and focus on what you need to do to survive.

Stay calm, bend your knees, and relax downwards.

The yin block

The yin block is a block that goes from outside the opponents arm inward towards the centre of your body. Usually the palm is up so that you are leading with the blade edge (ulna) of the forearm.

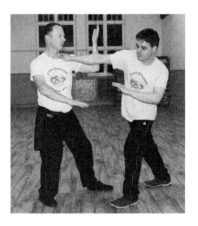

As soon as someone reaches forward to push or grab you sweep their arms to the side with the yin block. This will prevent them from continuing their attack with fist, knee or head as their body will be turned away from you. It is then easy for you to counter attack.

Eagle raises its wings

This defence is useful if someone grabs your clothes or even your throat with both hands. It involves raising both arms quickly under your opponent's arms thus knocking their arms upwards. From there you can quickly counter strike or take them down in a variety of ways. Once the wings have knocked his arms up, you could place your hands over his wrists and try to grab them. If you can then drop back into a cat stance and then lower your arms again. This will quickly pull him to the floor.

Beware. This is more powerful than you may think. If doing it to someone else for practice then do so carefully as it can easily cause whiplash type injuries when done at speed. If they don't go all the way down then raise the arm on the side of your forward foot and lower the other arm and twist your body. This should lever them down to the floor as shown below.

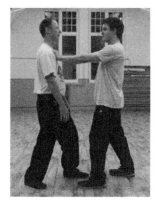

Opponent grabs or pushes

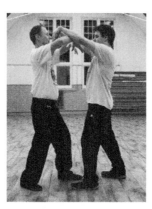

Raise forearms up sharply under opponent's arms

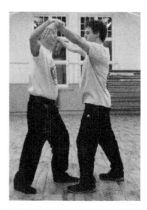

Place palms over his wrists and grab

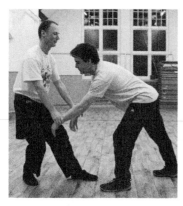

Drop elbows, drop back into cat stance and pull him down

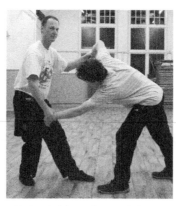

Raise left arm, lower right arm and start to twist to the right

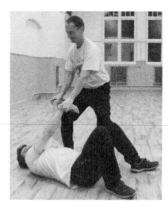

Turn to right in horse and lower opponent to the ground

Wrist pull down

This is another highly effective defence against being grabbed. If the opponent grabs you with his right hand place your own right hand over the back of his hand and wrap your middle two fingers around his wrist. Then lower your right elbow and use the elbow movement to pull his hand down. Keep your right hand facing left with your middle fingers around his wrist. This will twist his wrist and he will go down easily from the pain. The more relaxed into your stance you are the better this will work.

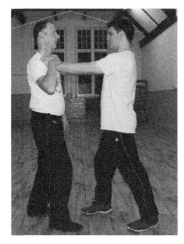

Place hand over opponent's hand and wrap middle finger around the wrist

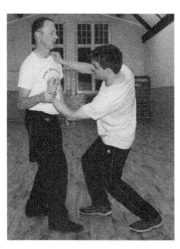

Relax your stance, drop your elbow and lead him downward

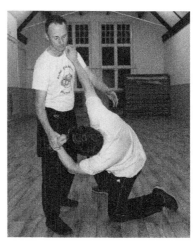

As he drops turn your grabbing hand out and push him onto his back with your spare hand

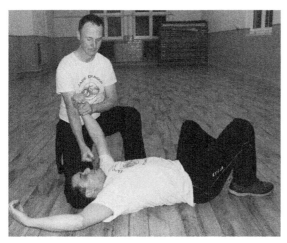

Control with locks or threaten him when he's down to prevent an attempt at counter-attack

Finally, don't forget that if someone is grabbing you then you are within their striking distance but equally they are within yours. It may be a good idea to strike their grabbing arm or their chest. Not too hard but enough to let them know you mean business and could strike harder if they persist.

Defences against grabs from behind

Being grabbed from behind can be frightening and very dangerous. If you are grabbed around the throat your attacker can cut off your air supply or the blood supply going to your head. Either of these could leave you quickly unconscious so you have to move fast.

Being grabbed from behind is dangerous so you must move quickly.

If you have been grabbed around the throat and are having trouble breathing you need to restore your air supply. Don't bother trying to pull their arm away as you won't have the strength. Instead place both hands over the crook of their elbow and push down. This will release the pressure enough to enable you to breathe. Now you need to release their grip. As they are in a strong position and behind you your options are limited. Try kicking back into their shins or back elbowing or even back headbutting them. All of these can work. At the top of your opponent's forearm, near the elbow joint is a muscle. Dig your fingertips hard into the muscle and that should produce a pain sharp enough to make them let go. Alternatively reach behind and grab them at the top of the leg just below the hip and dig your thumb in. The surprise coupled with pain will make most people jump back to get out of the way of it.

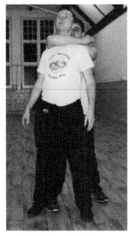
Opponent grabs from behind

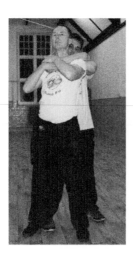
If you can't breathe push his elbow down to restore airway

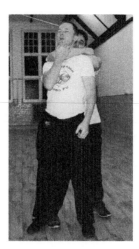
Dig fingers into the top of his forearm

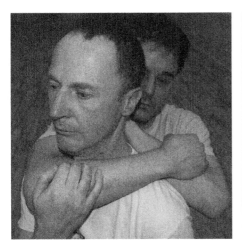

Close-up of fingers into forearm.

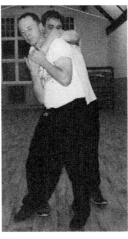

The pain of this will cause him to release

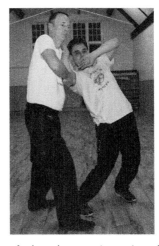

As he releases step outward into a position where you can counter

Another alternative is to throw your opponent over your shoulder. This is easier than it sounds. If he is grabbing you with his right arm then push his elbow down as you did to release your airway, drop onto your right knee, and lean forward. Don't step forward first just put your right knee next to or behind your left foot. This will put you under his centre of gravity and, as you lean forward, he will have to fall over your right shoulder.

Finally, and perhaps easiest of all just pinch his skin at the bottom of his upper arm. This sudden and unexpected pain will feel like a bee sting and he'll quickly let go. As always, the unpredictable technique is more likely to succeed than the predictable one.

Chapter 20.
Defences Against Strikes

Different people tend to punch in different ways. A boxer will punch in a different way to a karateka who will differ to an untrained person. You should be able to tell by the way a person moves or stands before striking what kind of fighter they are. As I have already said, if you believe you are about to be punched you should extend your arms forward to control the space between your opponent and yourself. This can be done in a non-threatening way by holding them with palms forward. Then, if a punch does fly your way, you can redirect it or cover it with either yin or yang blocks.

Yang blocks are your power blocks. They use an unbendable arm attached to a strong structure so they stop an incoming attack dead. He is literally striking at an immovable structure. Most people's bodies collapse on impact which is what he will be expecting so he would be in for a big surprise. Usually your block will land on the inside of your opponent's forearm which is the weakest part of his arm. If the block is good he will be in a great deal of pain, in fact the harder he punches you the more pain he will be in. Hopefully, so much that he won't be tempted to try it again. This is something my students know full well. When practicing the blocking and shielding skills they learn to pull their punches somewhat as it's simply too painful not to.

You should never rely on just a block on its own no matter how strong and painful to the opponent it may be.

Your block should always be accompanied by a strike with your other arm or some other technique. You could use either a yin or yang block followed by a dragon or tiger punch or any other punch of your choice. Also, when you block try to circle your opponent's arm around and down. This enables you to potentially grab his arm while circling and the downward force of the circle helps prevent him from following up with a kick, or almost any other technique. As his arm is being circled down it is more than likely that his body will bend forward to follow it. This makes him vulnerable to a wide range of locks and strikes.

Every move you make is not just controlling your opponent but also aims to limit what he can do next. This makes his next moves predictable and therefore easy to control. Although having said that you shouldn't allow him to make another move. You should always aim to keep the upper hand by maintaining control of the opponent and anticipating and preventing his counter-attacks. Naturally, if your own punch gets blocked and circled down you shouldn't let your body lean forward to follow it.

Getting close to an opponent is often safer than keeping a distance.

If your aim is to get close to your opponent, which is often a good idea with those who punch, then the yin block is a better bet. With this block, you aren't stopping his arm dead but redirecting it while you slip past it to get in close. With a yin block you can block with either the palm of your hand or the blade of the forearm. The yang circle is always done the same way but the yin circle is very adaptable. At the top and bottom position the hands can be facing each other ie upper hand palm down and lower hand palm up. In this position, your upper hand can close into a fist to strike with the thumb edge of the fist. This is a good way to strike someone on the side of the head. There is less chance of you breaking your hand or wrist with this strike than there is with the more typical punch using the front of the fist. It is also possible to perform this punch from further away as you don't need to bend your elbow and wrist to get the fist in position.

The other way to do the yin circle if for the hands to be facing away from each other ie upper hand palm up and lower hand palm down. With this variation, you are leading the move with the blades of the forearm so it is ideal for blocking all manner of attacks.

A final alternative for the yin circle is for your upper hand to be held with the palm to the side and the fingers pointing up to enable you to block with your palm. The lower hand would be held palm down to enable better blocks of kicks.

The yin circle enables you to get close to your opponent and use locks and throws to render them harmless. With the yin circle you block their incoming attack and try to maintain contact with it while you bend your elbow and move forward into throwing range. This can be done in a split second, all you need do is control their arm long enough to take a step forward. Then you may be in a position to try one of the throws mentioned earlier.

Joint locks give you control without causing damage.

As a general rule yang blocks work best for roundhouse style punches whereas yin blocks tend to work better for straight punches but it doesn't matter that much. There are no hard and fast rules in combat. The laws of most countries state that you shouldn't use excessive force to defend yourself. But if somebody strikes you then you could strike them back followed with a joint lock to control them if you feel competent enough to do so and the circumstances allow. Joint locks are great for self-defence as they give you control over your opponent but they don't do him any physical damage. You can control what he does with his body and also how much pain he is in. If he doesn't comply you can make the movement more painful. Nothing gets damaged apart from his ego. When you let go then 99% of his pain will go as well.

Another possibility, which is more useful for multiple attackers, is to use the chain punch where you can overwhelm them physically and mentally with a rapid-fire series of strikes to their arms and body. None of these strikes may do much, if any damage but the combined effect will be enough to put most attackers to the floor or running for their life.

Chapter 21.
Defences Against Kicks

In this section, I'm talking primarily about high kicks i.e. kicks aimed above waist height. Many combat sports use such kicks as their primary weapon. They argue that the legs are stronger than the arms so kicks are stronger than punches. We've already seen that this isn't necessarily the case. High kicks are fine if all you want to do is score points in a ring or impress some no-nothing who's giving you a hard time. They are not fine if you are facing a trained opponent in a real-life situation. They are also not fine if you happen to be wearing clothes that are a bit tight or are not warmed up properly. In the first case, you'd tear your clothes and in the second you're likely to tear your own muscles. However, it's possible that you may face someone who has trained such kicks and wants to use them on you. They are usually easy to spot. They will be restless on their feet, usually making small shuffling and jumping moves while waiting for an opportunity to kick. If you think somebody is going to kick you don't stand still. It is quite hard to kick a moving target and most kickers won't risk using their kicks unless they are pretty sure they will land on target.

Kickers also require a certain amount of space for their kicking skills to work so if you can close the gap and get close to them they will lose that advantage. When you are close you can use strikes, throws or joint locks to prevent them kicking you again. Tactically it is best to move forward to the outside of their forward foot. This is the area they will find it most difficult to kick into. So, if they're forward on their left leg step out with your right foot to the outside of their left foot. If you extend your left arm out at the same time you can grab them with it and be in a great position to throw.

All the throws that were covered in the throws section will work against kickers. People who kick are on one leg and their centre of balance tends to be high making them unstable and easy to throw down. One tactic we use is to step under the kicking leg. When somebody kicks, they assume they will be able to put their foot down where they choose. You can prevent this by stepping into a horse stance under their raised leg. This forces them to turn away from you and unbalances them by making their kicking leg slide down the outside of your horse stance. From here they are easy to push backwards and they'll hopefully fall over your horse stance. Their leg is forced to go forward and across their body while you push their torso backwards. They will fall at your feet so be sure to control them when they are down by keeping hold of their arm or keeping your arms and knees ready to cover any potential kicks or arm movements they might make.

High kicks such as roundhouse kicks can be caught with your elbows or the blades of your forearm (ulna). The yin circle is excellent for this as your two arms can circle out to the side and will trap their leg in a scissor movement. Obviously if you can catch a kick on your elbows, which isn't easy, it would be devastating for the kicker. This is why a lot of moves such as elbow blocks are illegal in combat sports. However, real life isn't a combat sport and if someone wants to attack you with moves they've learned in the ring and you defend yourself with what they would consider an illegal move that's their lookout. If you do manage to block their leg then give them a tap in the groin with your foot and you can be pretty sure they won't try it a second time.

Another option with kickers is to attack the legs themselves. Kickers value their legs, after all they need one of them to stand on while the other is used as a weapon. If you can damage or hurt either leg it's likely they won't have much else to offer.

Chapter 22.
Defences Against Grapplers

All grapplers learned their skills in combat sports, whether it be judo, wrestling or BJJ. All combat sports have rules and grapplers, like other participants in sports, aren't used to defending themselves against skills that are out of their rulebook. The biggest problem grapplers have with trying to use their skills in street fights is getting within clinching distance of their opponent. Many grappling sports like wrestling or judo start off in a clinch and it's then down to the skill of the fighter to take the other down first. Real life conflict isn't that easy. The grappler has to move in past kicking and striking range to be close enough to grab their opponent.

Grapplers don't train in standing practice in the way that most traditional Chinese martial arts do. They aren't used to aligning their whole body with the flow of gravity and using it to stick them firmly onto mother earth. Therefore, they also aren't used to grappling people who do. I have had several students of grappling styles as students and they all find it very difficult indeed to take their fellow students down. Indeed, with good stance training they will find it difficult to move you let alone take you to the floor successfully. Just be aware of your line of power - that is if you drew a line between your feet that is the direction in which you are strong. Any force applied perpendicular to that line will mean you have to move your feet into a different stance to stay strong. Often, it's simply a question of taking a small step backwards or forwards to keep your head over your hips and your hips over your feet. If your assailant or partner manages to upset this arrangement of head over hips over feet then you go from being very strong to being very vulnerable instantly. Again, find a partner and practice trying to throw each other or even push each other around and learn to change stances to keep yourself in a balanced and strong position. My more senior students are all but impossible for even me to take them down. They are too rooted in their stances, they maintain good alignments and are quick to move out of unfavourable positions. But do be aware that some grapplers will try to physically lift you off the ground to upset your root before taking you down. However, the defences that follow will prevent that from happening.

If someone is trying to get into grappling range with you then use the yang circle to keep them at bay. Whereas the yin circle will let you close the gap, the yang circle and its use of the unbendable arm principle is good at preventing others entering the zone between your arms in front of your body. In MMA grapplers get in close by going under their opponent's arms and clinching around the waist. If anyone should try this to you then they are in for an unpleasant surprise as you aren't bound by the rules of MMA. Feel free to break those MMA rules by driving your elbow down onto their back, feel equally free to grab their ears and twist or punch them in the back of the head. Maintain a good stance and they will have to literally lift you in the air to throw you down. The more upright and downwardly relaxed you are the harder they will find this. This will give you time for your counter-attack. Then they won't be holding on for long.

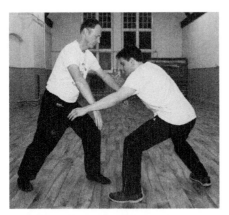

Use lower yang and yin blocks to keep an opponent from grabbing you down low

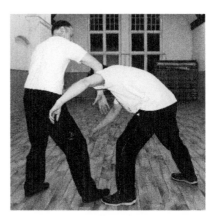

A lower yin block to the side of the head will be enough to knock them to the ground. A hard strike will knock them out

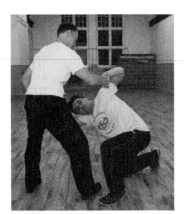

As they go down they can be controlled with their arms

A quick reminder about ground fighting is necessary here. Many martial arts are teaching ground fighting techniques and claiming them to be an essential part of any martial artist's repertoire. Ground-fighting may work in the ring or cage but is too dangerous for the street. Too many street fight situations involve more than just one man on one man and no amount of ground fighting techniques can prepare you for several guys kicking you while you're down. If you should happen to go to the ground you have only one priority and that is to get up again as soon as possible. Your stance training should make it difficult for anyone to take you down with joint locks or throws. But never, ever go to the floor voluntarily.

Chapter 23.
Defences Against Multiple
Attackers

This leads me onto the thorny problem of dealing with multiple attackers. This is not an uncommon scenario in the street yet is an area that is rarely, if ever, covered in most martial arts classes. This is because almost all martial arts are firmly focused on one man on one man. To be able to cope with more than one attacker means changing your tactics as well as some fundamental things about the way you perform your martial arts.

The first and possibly most important thing you need to change is your focus. In all combat sports and most martial arts training you can, and indeed should focus all your attention on the man or woman in front of you. This is possible because you know nobody else is going to try and attack you at the same time. You know there are no obstacles in the way of your movement. You know there are no implements you or he could grab to use as weapons. Clearly in real life street conflict this is a luxury you cannot afford. You need to widen your awareness to take in your environment be alert as to how it could help or hinder you. If you are indoors where are the exits and what route can you take to get there quickly? If you're outside are there any obstacles you can put between yourself and your assailant? Are there any onlookers who may get involved in the action? These and a thousand other possibilities depending on the circumstances should be on your mind. You also need to be aware of yourself. Are you wearing tight clothes that might restrict your movements? Are you tense in the wrong places, are you breathing high in the chest or are you able to bend your knees, sink your weight and your breath and so make yourself better able to deal with the conflict?

As I mentioned earlier if you can gain and maintain physical contact with your assailant then you don't need to look at him and can look around you to be aware of other opportunities or threats. This need for a greater awareness of environment leads us onto the next important point for training against multiple attacks

Kung fu is largely taught through the learning of forms. Each form consists of movements that move the whole body through forward, backward or sideways steps and turns of the waist. It is these stepping and turning patterns that give you whole body power but they also give you something else. They enable you to look around you in different directions to be aware of changes in your environment. If your feet are side by side you can see what is in front of you and to ninety degrees left and right. If you step forward on your right foot you can see more of what is on your left side and part of what is behind you. If you add turns of the waist and hips you increase your range of vision even more. Start to use the stepping and twisting movements of your forms to be able to maintain a continuous survey of your environment even while you are performing your martial movements. This will make it all but impossible for an attacker to sneak up on you and take you by surprise.

You have now improved your overall awareness and can use your movements to enable you to maintain a constant survey or what's going on around you. However, you are being threatened by a small group of guys. What tactics can you use to minimise the danger to yourself and get out of there in one piece?

One tactic we practice in my classes is the human shield. To do this well does require knowledge of how to control someone through their wrists and elbows. Basically, you take control of one attacker and manipulate him to keep him between yourself and the other attacker. This does only really work well if you are threatened by two men. Any more than that and you can't use the human shield to defend yourself against more than one at a time. It is good fun to practice though!

Essentially, when dealing with multiple attackers, you need genuine battlefield tactics. This means you should be able to take one opponent down quickly and decisively while staying aware as to what is going on around you. The whole point of learning effortless power is to enable you to dispose of an opponent without undue effort. You cannot afford to waste any more time or energy on each opponent than necessary. Effortless power enables you take someone down with the smallest of moves and move quickly onto the next attacker. This is also where good, functional forms training is essential. It takes many years to master adaptable form movements using effortless power but all kung fu training is leading up to it.

It takes a long time and lots and lots of effort to make kung fu truly effortless.

I hope you have enjoyed this book. You can now see that kung fu is deeper than other martial arts with wider ranging benefits. Kung fu training empowers you in so many ways. It creates a healthy mind and body and teaches you to deal with the physical and emotional effects of stress. It contains an enormous range of skills, exercises, principles, philosophies and esoteric practices. It is a path you can walk for the whole of your life without ever getting tired or bored.

But remember, above all else, kung fu means PRACTICE.

Afterword

The eight animal styles

I teach a system that contains eight animal styles. I am writing more books to be published after this one which will introduce the reader to these animal styles. They will be a follow up to this book so it's essential that you train your body using the exercises in this book first. To whet your appetite here is an article I wrote that introduces you to the eight animal styles I teach.

Have you ever been inspired to walk through life with the confident power of a tiger or to achieve the tranquil balance of a crane or the playful agility of a monkey? If so you certainly wouldn't be alone.

The animal kung fu styles of China have long held a fascination for many. Incredible legends have been woven about the exploits of animal kung fu Masters. Stories have been written about them and films, even cartoons, made.

Some of the most famous kung fu styles have been based on the movements of animals. The Chinese of old admired the beauty, power, grace and fluidity of various animals and sought to emulate them. They copied their movements and their fighting tactics and created some of the most beautiful and deadly martial arts the world has ever seen.

Training in the animal kung fu styles brought to the student the qualities of that animal so that you would become more like the animal whose style you were studying. Each animal would also develop certain physical and personality traits within the student such as patience, aggression, fluidity of movement, awareness of environment, playfulness and so on.

The Shaolin Legend

In the traditional legends of the Shaolin temple it is said that the monks there originally learned exercises from five animals - the tiger, monkey, leopard, snake, and dragon. These exercises were given to strengthen the bodies of the monks who had been sitting all day in meditation. These five animals have lived on in kung fu legend and now many other animals styles are practised around the world. In the Jade Dragon kung fu tradition that I teach, we study eight animal kung fu styles. These are the original five of tiger, monkey, leopard, snake and dragon plus the crane, the mantis and the eagle.

There are many different variations of each of the animals taught in different schools so the knowledge that is briefly described here may not be the same as is taught in other kung fu traditions.

Please note that the information below refers only to my teachings and interpretations of the animal styles. Each school will interpret the animals in different ways.

All martial arts styles, whether they are aware of it or not specialise in just one element of combat. No school can teach you everything you need to know to be an all-round fighter no matter how much they claim otherwise. For example, judo specialises in taking the opponent to the ground and keeping him there. Karate was developed to defend against armed samurai attacking on horseback hence the high kicks to dismount the samurai and the powerful punches to smash through their bamboo armour. Each art deals with a particular aspect of combat and usually works best under certain circumstances.

I teach eight styles - hence eight different elements of combat are covered. Here is a brief overview of those eight animal styles.

Tiger style

Once the Jade Dragon student is familiar with the fundamental skills, which are partially covered in this book, the tiger style is the first style to be learned.

The tiger is a hugely powerful animal with no natural predators. When attacking it uses relatively simple moves and relies on its weight and raw physical strength. It applies that strength directly with little in the way of evasion or tactics, preferring to go through rather than around an opponent.

The tiger style is most suited to physically strong individuals and enables them to channel that power. However, that doesn't mean that less powerful people can't benefit from it. It is particularly beneficial to learn early on in training as it develops the ability to relax your upper body down into your stance and to use weighted power to overcome an assailant. There are no complicated movements to learn, it's mostly about developing strong yet fluid muscles and using gravity and connected movements rather than inefficient, localised force.

On a wider note the tiger style develops the ability to attack directly the root of the problem without over analysing every aspect of the situation.

Key benefits:

- Develops physical power

- Develops great rooting power

- Movements aren't complicated to learn.

- Eventually teaches fine muscle control, the ability to relax or tense individual muscles at will

Crane style

The crane is a long-range animal style especially suited to tall practitioners with long limbs. It uses sweeping movements of the arms to clear a way through attacks and lock or throw an attacker along with striking movements of the beak on vital parts of the body. This is combined with comprehensive kicking patterns as the crane is used to standing on one leg. Studying the crane is a study in angles of attack and defence.

The crane will stand in a studied pose until the prey comes within range then hop out of the way, defend and counter attack from many unusual angles then patiently stand on one leg waiting for the prey to come within range again. It's kicks and wing strikes are capable of breaking bones and damaging joints easily. This is because the crane is an expert in balance. The more balanced you are physically and mentally the more power you are able to focus with your body. Being out of balance even slightly will prevent part of your body and mind being involved in your movement skills as they will be occupied in keeping you upright.

Key benefits:

- It teaches strength through postural alignments

- Develops an understanding of biomechanics and leverage

- Patience, balance and the ability to extend force in many directions.

- Kicking skills and sophisticated use of knee and elbow blocks and strikes

Leopard style

Among African big game hunters, the leopard is considered to be the most dangerous animal they can face (despite the fact that the hippo kills more people). This is because unlike a lion, when faced by a group of men the leopard won't fix its attention on one man and maul only him but will leap from one man to the next killing or severely mauling each in rapid succession. It is also said that the leopard is the only animal, apart from man, that will kill for fun.

The leopard style is one of the most useful when faced with multiple attackers due to its sheer ferocity and speed. It rapidly moves from one man to the next delivering rapid fire strikes and kicks, often not bothering to block but directly hitting the incoming attacks with the famed leopard paw strikes. It is the most ferocious of the animal styles and so is useful in bringing out the 'killer instinct' in usually passive people.

Key benefits:

- Develops speed of attack
- Develops fearlessness and the ability to attack without warning and without mercy
- Uses a light root so that it can remain quick footed
- Probably the most effective system for dealing with multiple attackers

Monkey style

The monkey is the most agile of animals with arms as strong as its legs. It leaps and rolls then grabs and strikes with amazing rapidity. It is a playful creature that taunts its prey then comes in under an attack and uses short range strikes and throws often rolling over the opponent when he's on the floor.

The monkey is an expert at bringing an opponent in and taking him down while striking with multiple attacks and kicks. It treats its opponent as a tree that it wants to climb. It pulls them down and uses all manner of elbows, knees and fist strikes to attack. It also likes to get in close and use leverage to apply very powerful joint locks and throws.

Its speed, unpredictability, and ground fighting techniques make it a difficult style to counter.

Key benefits:

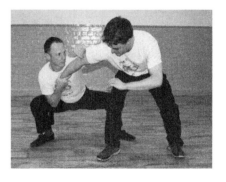

- Physically demanding style to learn
- Develops contractive power,
- Agility and mobility even when crouching down
- Strength in the arms and hands.

Eagle style

Many people have heard of the eagle claw style but eagle claw doesn't make full use of the eagle's wing movements. These powerful arm movements provide the eagle with superb defensive skills.

The eagle shares some similarities with the crane but where the crane is a ground fighting bird, the eagle attacks while in flight. The eagle's wings are powerful but sensitive enough to detect small changes in air pressure or an attacker's movements. The eagle's powerful talons are used to lock or strike the opponent and the general movement of the eagle's enormously powerful wings keep it covered from attacks from all directions, sweeping them out of the way and opening the opponent to talon and wing strikes.

The eagle is a yang animal. It expands its wings out and its mind and intention with them. The eagle style has one of the best defences of any kung fu style I've seen. Many of our arm movements that are covered in this book such as the yin circle and yang circle are derived from eagle wing movements. The eagle mind (covered in book three) develops the ability to become far more aware of your environment and to be able to deal with attacks from multiple directions.

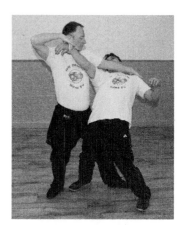

Key benefits:

- Develops power in extended arm movements.

- Has probably the best defensive skills of all the animals

- Develops a heightened sensitivity to your environment and the ability to rise above situations, thus avoid getting bogged down in the details.

Snake style

The snake is unique among our animals in having no legs. This means it cannot use strong stances so instead it develops power through coiling movements of the waist, legs and upper body.

The snake is a yin animal, cold, able to use constrictive power and able to penetrate the strongest and most complicated defence. The snake coils itself around the attacker in many different ways then strikes with extreme speed penetrating muscle, sinew and organ at weak points of the body. As a cold-blooded animal, it spends most of its time conserving its energy in enclosed spaces. It doesn't look for trouble but is capable of bringing down and consuming animals much larger than it is. At the highest level, it is the most instantly lethal of all the animals.

Key benefits:

- Develops the ability to find the gaps in any defence and strike with precision.

- Opens all the joints to enable coiling, wave like movements through the body and limbs.

- Teaches balance and patience, waiting for the prey to come within range.

- The snake develops the yin qualities of moving with the whole body and striking with whip-like power

Mantis style

The mantis style is, in many ways similar to the monkey style. It is a short-range system that uses complicated footwork with elbows and finger strikes to hit vital pressure points. The mantis, being an insect, has no higher thoughts and is all instinct and reflex. The mantis style which I teach differs from other mantis styles and is specialised at close range fighting. The Tang-Lang style which mixes mantis with monkey footwork is reputed to be the only system that defeated the monks of Shaolin.

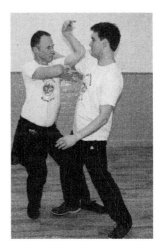

Key benefits:

- Speed and patience

- Best style for close range fighting

- Teaches anatomical knowledge of pressure point targets

- Fast reflexes

- Sophisticated use of elbows and knees

Dragon style

The Jade Dragon kung fu system is so called for very good reasons. The dragon is the animal that most represents the principles on which the system is based.

The Chinese Dragon is symbolic of the Chinese character. It is not a single animal as such but an entity composed of the most diverse creatures - the horse, eagle, ox, snake, deer and fish. The Chinese dragon is associated with water and so the dragon style uses flowing, twisting and coiling movements as if it were moving in water. These movements, similar to the snakes, generate force through the whole body and through every movement and angle of attack and defence. The dragon's movements are circular and they follow the movements of its opponent, quickly finding their weaknesses and instantly counter attacking with smooth power. Fighting a dragon is like being overwhelmed by a huge wave or being sucked into a whirlpool and drowned. It has a wide range of locks, throws, strikes and so on and the coiling footwork and body help the dragon to move in and out of dangerous situations and attack from many angles.

You cannot fight water as you cannot apply force directly to it, it moves out of the way and the dragon style does the same.

Key benefits:

- Develops power in every part of the body

- Opens the joints for increased qi flow

- The dragon style is usually the last style to learn as it draws on and brings together elements of each of the other seven animals.

Training in a variety of animal kung fu styles makes you a more rounded person by strengthening your weaknesses and developing your abilities in many different areas. The wide range of movements you can learn in a school such as the Jade Dragon school will make it so much easier to learn other physical skills such as other sports or dance etc. You will develop power and patience, grace and speed, calmness of mind and a will of steel. To study one animal is a privilege - to study eight animals is an opportunity that very few outsiders to the closed world of real Chinese martial arts will ever gain.

In the next book of this series I will go over the principles of good kung fu. I will show you in more detail how to put your entire body weight into any part of your body for true whole-body power. I will discuss the natural energy that the Chinese call chi and how to develop it as well as clear up the many misunderstandings about it. I will also introduce you to four of the animals from the system I teach: the tiger, leopard, monkey and crane. The other four animals will be introduced in the third book of this series.

If you have enjoyed this book then check out the online training section of our school website www.jadedragonschool.com. On there you will find videos on many of the skills found in this book along with other new articles and videos which are being added all the time.

Index

abdominal breathing......................154

abdominal exercises.........................91

abdominal muscles..........................86

acrobatic 14, 17

adaptability13, 17, 18, 19, 20, 21, 30, 51, 58, 64, 173

aggression.....................13, 28, 56, 160

aikido 14, 117, 140

All-China Wushu Association............37

animal stylesxi, xii, 5, 34, 131, 182, 183, 185

attitude..........................25, 26, 56, 160

awareness...49, 127, 152, 180, 181, 182

back kick............68, 135, 137, 138, 139

back muscles 48, 71, 72, 89, 93, 135

baguazhang 5, 36, 37, 55, 152

balance8, 19, 47, 48, 49, 51, 66, 67, 71, 81, 82, 83, 89, 93, 94, 95, 97, 104, 108, 111, 120, 121, 122, 131, 134, 136, 137, 138, 140, 146, 157, 159, 164, 175, 182, 184, 187

black belt 56

Bodhidharma..................................34

bodyweight training.........................84

boxers guard 116

breath8, 14, 49, 61, 62, 66, 67, 88, 125, 154, 180

Bruce Lee.......................1, 21, 38, 124

Buddhism 34

Buddhist 34, 35, 48

cardiovascular training.....................96

cat step.............................109, 110, 111

cat to dragon step...........................109

chain punch.............131, 132, 133, 174

chambering.....................................79

Chen family 16

chi...152

children 18, 22

circular movement 102, 116, 151

circular training.............................102

combat sports...................................55

combat variables..............................25

common types of assault.................165

complete martial art 50, 51

Confucian 43, 59, 73

Confucianism 34

contracts.....................................11, 57

coordination 8, 52, 67, 68, 84, 150

countering14, 22, 29, 108, 128, 134, 143, 158, 164, 166, 167, 173, 178, 184, 185, 187

crane stance 135

crane style 184

Cultural Revolution.....................38, 41

Da Mo 34

dantian 93

David Carradine 38

defences against grabs....................167

dit da jow......................................125

dragon punch 122, 128, 129, 130

dragon step....................................107

dragon style....................................187

dragon throw 145

dynamic stretching 98

eagle raises its wings.......................167

eagle style.....................................185

effortless powerxiii, 4, 8, 9, 14, 43, 71, 72, 73, 149, 151, 181

energyxiv, 8, 11, 14, 16, 48, 51, 66, 83, 84, 97, 99, 104, 112, 152, 154, 158, 161, 181, 186, 188

experimentation3, 13, 16, 41, 42, 43, 44, 68, 72, 102, 122

extended guard ....ix, 112, 113

fajin.. 15
fight or flight reflex.......................... 13
five animal kung fu.......................... 182
flexibilityxiv, 8, 14, 18, 52, 63, 64, 65, 96, 97, 98, 99, 102, 103, 126, 134, 135
flying crane 93, 94
formsxii, 1, 3, 13, 17, 18, 19, 20, 21, 22, 23, 26, 28, 30, 37, 41, 52, 58, 64, 65, 80, 180
    as a learning aid............................ 20
    fully functional 17, 18, 19, 22
    partly functional................ 17, 18, 21
    stylised form 17, 18
four levels..8
front kick 135, 136, 137, 139
generic training.............. 4, 7, 39, 63, 64
grabs from behind........................... 170
Grandmaster..................................... 59
grappling49, 114, 119, 141, 156, 165, 177
gravity52, 74, 75, 77, 82, 84, 97, 98, 107, 110, 141, 142, 145, 151, 156, 171, 183
ground fighting141, 142, 144, 178, 185, 186
ground path 75
half dragon step 107, 108
half tiger step 108
hand conditioning 124
hand-to-hand combat...........................9
hard and soft tension...................97, 98
healing 10
high kicks 134
Hip and Shoulder Opener 100
history of kung fu2, 3, 15, 16, 32, 33, 38, 39, 41, 44
humility 61
hundred schools of thought 34
iron palm 125
iron shirt 15
Jade Dragonxii, xiii, 6, 22, 109, 114, 128, 137, 182, 183, 187, 188
Japanese.. 37
judo 13, 35, 56
jujitsu 35, 57, 65, 156

karate 3, 13, 58, 65, 78
kicking.......................... 13, 30, 134, 135
kicks18, 21, 42, 64, 73, 111, 119, 135, 136, 137, 157, 163, 166, 173, 175, 176, 183, 184, 185
kung fu body 4, 63
kung fu levels 8
kyphosis 106
learning process.............................. 68
leg raises 91, 92
leopard style................................... 184
line of power............................. 77, 177
lineages 3, 37, 44, 45, 46
locks13, 50, 105, 119, 126, 138, 143, 145, 156, 157, 159, 172, 173, 175, 179, 185, 188
lower yang block 115
lower yin block 116
Manchus..................................... 14, 36
mantis style 187
MAP.......................... viii, 104, 106, 135
martial contracts 57
Master Irvine 5
meditation................. 5, 16, 34, 50, 182
mental health................................ 7, 48
mind5, 7, 8, 13, 14, 41, 50, 52, 61, 66, 67, 68, 123, 157, 161, 186, 188
mindfulness..................................... 49
Ming dynasty 35, 36
MMA.......................... 3, 119, 177
monkey style 185
move from the centre...................... 151
multiple attackers42, 56, 156, 174, 180, 181, 184, 185
multiple discovery 16
Nanjing Central Guoshu Institute ... 36
neijia.. 35, 39
obesity 96
obliques 91
panic.. x, 154
panic attack 154
partnerx, 18, 21, 29, 30, 69, 73, 75, 105, 107, 116, 117, 119, 132, 140, 142, 143, 145, 158, 161, 162, 163, 177

passive stretching 98

philosophyxiii, 7, 9, 13, 15, 16, 34, 38, 50, 124, 141

Pinyin xiii

posture........65, 85, 87, 96, 97, 122, 158

potential energy 150

power breaking.......................124, 131

power movements 149

press-ups...............57, 84, 85, 87, 88, 89

Pressure points 50

pressure testing19, 56, 69, 72, 73, 76, 78, 107

principlesxiii, 5, 6, 7, 8, 9, 15, 16, 19, 21, 30, 39, 42, 43, 48, 58, 73, 74, 76, 105, 149, 154, 157, 162, 163, 165, 187, 188

proof..24

pullups...89, 90

push hands 27, 127, 158, 162

qigong 5, 6, 11, 50

Qing dynasty 36, 39

range of movement87, 97, 98, 101, 102, 150

reaction speed.......................25, 26, 161

reflexes.................67, 75, 125, 127, 187

relax downwards 138, 154, 155, 167

resisting opponents..19, 24, 28, 29, 157

reverse chain punch..........................133

rooting42, 60, 75, 102, 108, 110, 120, 123, 130, 135, 136, 138, 140, 142, 152, 157, 162, 164, 166, 177, 183, 185

rules of engagement.....................25, 26

sacrifice throws 141

self-defence 2, 4, 135, 143, 153, 173

sensitivity 52, 66, 124, 125, 127, 186

Shaolin.............32, 34, 35, 36, 182, 187

shield 112, 113, 166, 181

Sifu...59

Sino-Japanese war 37

snake style..186

sparringxii, 3, 5, 17, 19, 21, 24, 25, 26, 28, 29, 30, 40, 73, 131, 146

specific training2, 4, 10, 15, 17, 27, 28, 29, 33, 63, 64, 65, 66, 67, 108, 121, 131, 156, 165

squats 85, 87

  circular squats..............................87

  close squats....................................87

  uneven squats................................87

stamina.......................................96, 133

stancesvii, 1, 18, 19, 70, 71, 72, 73, 74, 75, 76, 77, 78, 79, 80, 81, 82, 83, 85, 86, 94, 103, 106, 107, 108, 109, 110, 111, 117, 119, 122, 123, 128, 129, 130, 133, 135, 136, 137, 138, 140, 142, 143, 145, 146, 147, 150, 156, 157, 159, 160, 162, 167, 169, 177, 178, 179, 183, 186

  cat stance 80, 81, 111

  crane stance.....................................81

  dragon stance77, 78, 107, 109, 140, 145, 158

  horse stance70, 72, 73, 74, 76, 79, 140, 145, 146, 175

  tiger stance 79, 80, 109

stay smooth 163

stepping movements 19

steroids 91

stop the fight 7

Stress Proof Your Bodyii, 6, 8, 48, 67, 155

stretching . 63, 65, 84, 86, 96, 97, 98, 99

strikes13, 73, 107, 123, 129, 131, 132, 133, 156, 157, 166, 172, 173, 174, 175, 184, 185, 186, 187, 188

structure14, 39, 41, 51, 52, 65, 67, 70, 104, 106, 107, 146, 172

t'ai chi.. 10

t'ai chi chuanxiii, 10, 12, 16, 18, 27, 32, 35, 36, 37, 42, 83, 123, 150, 152, 158, 162

tacticsxiii, 4, 14, 30, 33, 41, 51, 55, 153, 156, 159, 180, 181, 182, 183

taekwondo 3, 156

Taoism ....xiii, 9, 11, 34, 35, 38

Taoist 11, 16, 23, 34, 35, 48

technique sparring............................29

technique variables...............25, 27, 28

tensionxiv, 6, 8, 48, 49, 50, 51, 52, 61, 63, 65, 66, 69, 71, 74, 75, 82, 83, 84,

85, 86, 89, 93, 96, 97, 98, 99, 100, 101, 102, 104, 117, 120, 121, 127, 129, 145, 151, 154, 159, 160, 161

The Clock 101
three types of attacker 155
three types of martial arts 156
throws 13, 50, 73, 76, 140, 141, 142, 143, 145, 147, 156, 157, 165, 173, 175, 179, 185, 188
  backward horse throw 146
  dragon throw 143
  forward horse throw 145, 146
tiger punch 130, 172
tiger style 183
tiger to dragon step 109
timing 25, 28
traditional schools 28, 32, 38, 41, 46, 55
transfer your weight 150
turn the waist 150
unbendable arm 112, 114, 117, 118, 172, 177
upper yang block 114, 115
upper yin block 115
Wade-Giles system xiii
walking 110
warlords 15, 33, 36
weapons 9, 10, 50, 126, 128, 180
  broadsword 10

spear 10
staff 10, 17, 126
straight sword 10
weight training 14, 72, 84, 121
whole-body power xiv, 1, 14, 18, 19, 30, 42, 105, 106, 188
wing chun 1, 27, 55, 131, 133, 162
wirework 42
wrist pull down 168
wu 34
Wudang 35, 36, 37
wushu 2, 18, 37, 42
xingyiquan 36, 37
yang 14
  properties 11
Yang 11, 114, 172
yang circle 113, 116, 118, 119, 173, 177, 186
yin 12
  properties 11
Yin 11, 114, 119
yin and yang 10, 11, 12, 14
yin block .... x, 114, 147, 166, 167, 173
yin circle 105, 113, 119, 166, 173, 176, 177, 186
yoga 99
YouTube 15, 24, 28, 29, 51, 99, 105
Zhang Sanfeng 16, 35

Printed in Great Britain
by Amazon